Atlas of Cross-Sectional
Anatomy and Radiological Imaging

By
David J. Jackowe, MD

College of Charleston, Charleston, South Carolina
Formerly *University of Hawaii*

Illustrated by
David J. Jackowe, MD and Viktor Deak

Published by:

Anshan Ltd
6 Newlands Road
Tunbridge Wells
Kent. TN4 9AT

UK.

Tel: +44 (0) 1892 557767
Fax: +44 (0) 1892 530358

e-mail: info@anshan.co.uk
web site: www.anshan.co.uk

© 2013 Anshan Ltd

ISBN: 978 1 848290 570

British Library Cataloguing in Publication Data
A catalogue record for this book is available from the British Library.

Copy Editor: Andrew White
Cover Design: Emma Randall
Cover Image: David J Jackowe
Typeset by: Kerrypress Ltd, Luton, Bedfordshire

This Book is Dedicated to Special K

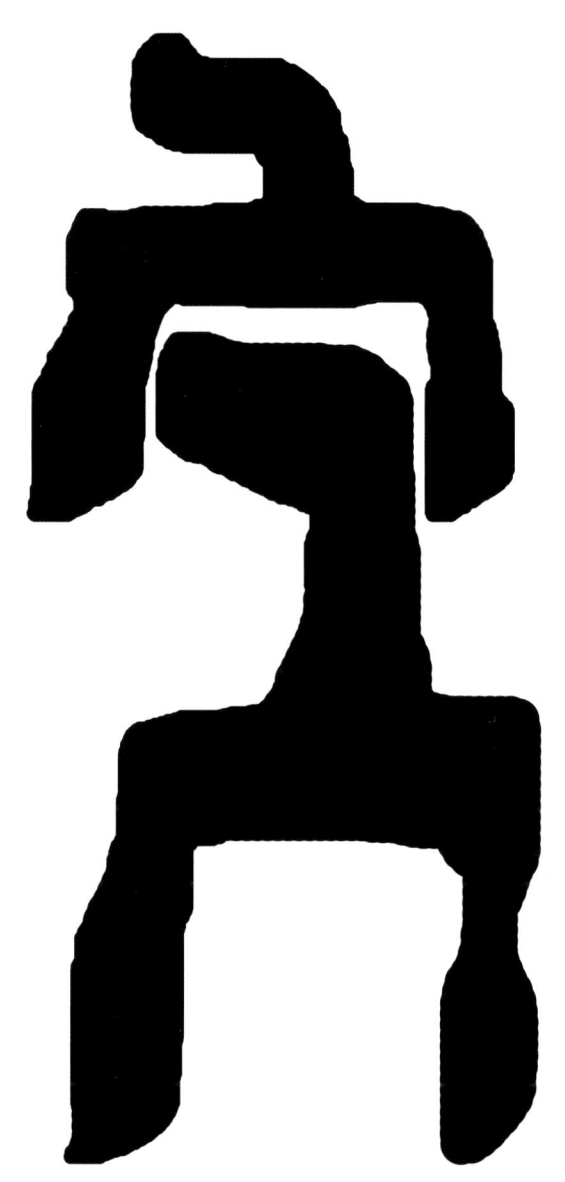

Contents

Introduction

On the place for anatomies which has recently been constructed at Amsterdam

Evil men, who did harm when alive, do good after their deaths:
Health seeks advantages from Death itself.

Dumb integuments teach. Cuts of flesh, though dead,
for that very reason forbid us to die.

Here, while with artful hand he slits the pallid limbs,
speaks to us the eloquence of learned Tulp:

"Listener, learn yourself! and while you proceed through the parts,
believe that, even in the smallest, God lies hid."

- Caspar Barlaeus

Maundy Thursday

Between the brown hands of a server-lad
The silver cross was offered to be kissed.
The men came up, lugubrious, but not sad,
And knelt reluctantly, half-prejudiced.
(And kissing, kissed the emblem of a creed.)
Then mourning women knelt; meek mouths they had,
(And kissed the Body of the Christ indeed.)
Young children came, with eager lips and glad.
(These kissed a silver doll, immensely bright.)
Then I, too, knelt before that acolyte.
Above the crucifix I bent my head:
The Christ was thin, and cold, and very dead:
And yet I bowed, yea, kissed – my lips did cling.
(I kissed the warm live hand that held the thing.)

- Wilfred Owen

This book is about perspective—a corporeal perspective and a poetic one. There are two problems in anatomy and medicine that I hope to address here. The first is this: Learning the proper sequence and orientation of axial cross-sections and CT scans is often extremely challenging, even for the most dedicated students. One reason for this is that the shapes seen in the axial plane have little relation to the more familiar coronal, and the gray-white patterns of CT slices are little more than the silhouettes of real organs. Most of the available textbooks are little help in this regard as they abandon students either to memorize the shapes seen at high-yield vertebral levels, or else perform tricky mental gymnastics as they mentally rotate the axial plane to the more familiar coronal.

This book tries to encourage the conceptual mastery of cross-sections and CT scans by presenting them as 3-Dimensional images. Here, the human body is shown from a three-quarters perspective. This unique angle allows the axial, coronal, and sagittal planes to be appreciated simultaneously, and the 3-Dimensional orientation of organs understood in the context of the body as a whole—rather than as 1-Dimensional shapes that are memorized and quickly forgotten.

But there is another problem, one, that at first may seem superficial, but with a bit of reflection is just as serious as not being able to conceptualize diagnostic images. The problem is the way modern textbooks nurture a perspective in which a human being is reduced to no more than a morphological specimen.

Consider this: For centuries, anatomy books were elaborately illustrated, as in the woodcut seen here, a tradition popularized by Andreas Vesalius in his 16th century atlas *De Humani Corporis Fabrica*. Just what were the old anatomists looking for when they peeled away that "slim covering of radiant skin over ugly organs?"[1] The aphorism *nosce te ipsum* appears in many classic anatomy illustrations and was also prominently displayed in dissection theatres. Meaning "know thyself," the phrase reflects the perception of anatomy as way to self-knowledge, both of the physical and transcendent self.[2] Vesalius captured this idea by the way the écorché, or muscle man, looks longingly to the heavens, beckoning god with one arm, while with his other he points to the earth. This is the human condition: the body, while believed to be a divine manifestation of the glory of god, is also ephemeral: "Those who have fallen in battle are beautiful but what when the dogs begin to dishonour the corpses?"[3] The use of realistic backgrounds further speaks to man's relationship with his environment. He is inseparable from the world in which he lives—nature and man are a co-existence. While teaching morphology was certainly important to Vesalius, the human being was never understood to be just a morphology, a collection of "dumb integuments." For many Humanists, the subject of anatomy books—the human being—could only be accurately illustrated both body and soul.

It may seem like nothing more than old superstition to go hunting for god in a dissection lab. But it is important to remember that the religious language used by the Renaissance anatomists is far from ecclesiastical. For many anatomists, the idea that god lies hid in the body represented an intellectual and spiritual curiosity about the human condition—god was the secret to the universe, the answer to the perennial question "What is this?" Living in a Christian era, these questions naturally took on religious language, and even today, the curiosity in man's heart has changed little except for the language used to express it. Just what is the holy-grail of modern science?

---

1 Balthazar, p. 23.
2 "Know thyself" is something of a paradox, a case of the snake swallowing its own tail, as the phrase implies that "the knower" and "what is known" are separate and distinct entities. In terms of perspective: Who cares?
3 Balthazar, p.53. An eloquent paraphrase of the Iliad.

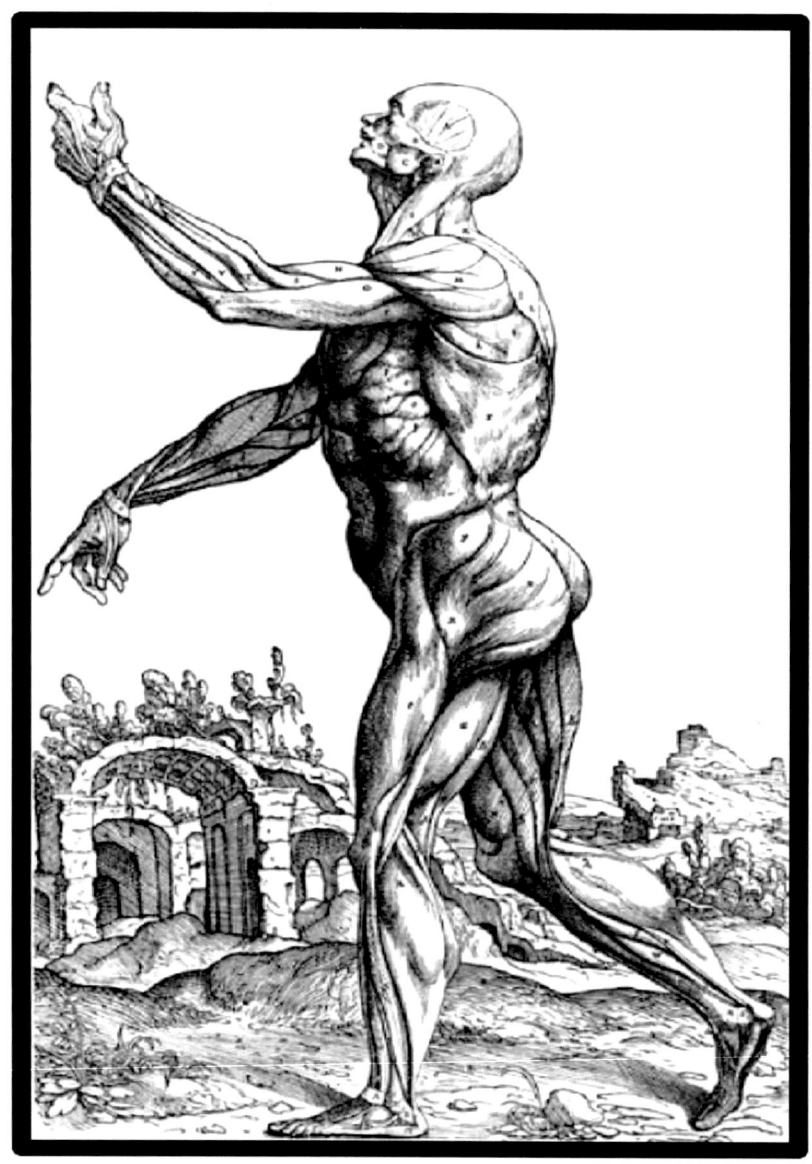

It used to be that a god's name contained his power, and to his followers it was holy because it represented the secret of the universe distilled down to a single word. As cultures changed with time and technology, so too did the names and personalities of their deities. This phenomenon continues even today. Consider quantum physics. As Roland Barthes writes of Albert Einstein, the famed physicist achieved mythological status because he awakened man's belief that the universe is a safe and he almost found its combination.[4] In many ways, the equation $E=mc^2$ is the secularist's tetragrammaton. It is god with another name, spoken in the language of science, the paradigm of the modern era. Whereas the philosophical concept of god can

4   Barthes, p. 69.

represent perfection, Einstein's equation, at best, can only come asymptotically close. Isn't a more perfect equation, the secret of the universe contained in a single word, what any curious scientist hopes to discover?

Over the past two centuries, anatomists have worked hard to rid themselves of the aesthetic of myth and religion. By the mid-nineteenth century, works such as Henry Gray's eponymous atlas represented the death of Humanism in anatomy.[5] With its emotionless figures and diagrams, Gray's book was certainly innovative in its treatment of human morphology. However, innovation can only be innovative for as long as the memory of what it replaced is actively remembered. Today, in the age of evidence based medicine, stories of humours and phlegms, of pneumas and spirits, of fig leaves and grave-robbers, are no more than the hobbies of emeritus faculty and rare book collectors. But a century-and-a-half ago, a time when a psychiatric patient was still thought to be under the control of the moon—he was, after all a *lun*atic— Gray understood that if medicine was ever going to be taken seriously, old superstitions had to be replaced with the scientific method. Anatomy books changed to reflect the attitude of the empiricists, and soon, the living men and women who graced the pages of Vesalius, Estienne, and Casserio in lively vivisection became utilitarian diagrams—morphologies. Such was the god shaped hole cut out of the cadaver. For generations since students have learned from books in which a man was a "silver doll," a well-crafted, anatomically precise "emblem of a creed."

If this was any other science than medicine, none of this would matter much, save for the loss felt by a sentimental or romantic few. But if physicians are serious when they say that a person is more than just morphology plus pathology, shouldn't a more Humanist aesthetic be presented in textbooks? How can students be expected to pass through medical school, reading nothing but books filled with flow charts, decision trees, and diagrams of man-as-machine and not lose their soul—not acquire the perspective that man *is* his morphology?

This book is the first text produced in years that attempts to recreate a classic Humanist aesthetic. This is neither atavism, nor a new-age gripe with medical science. Rather, a profession that advertises itself as valuing compassion—whatever that word may mean—cannot reasonably expect to encourage any sort of genuine emotion if it relies on sterile science books to shape its students' perspectives of humanity. Science does many wonderful things; but one thing it cannot do is teach a student that a human being is anything other than a silver doll. In this book, I have designed each illustration in the Humanist spirit so that students can learn the science of anatomy without forgetting that the whole point of their education is that there is "a warm live hand." It is my hope that readers will find that these illustrations have successfully combined the Humanist aesthetic with all the knowledge of modern science.

Just as being inundated with sterile diagrams can inadvertently result in students acquiring the perspective of man as morphology, so too can speaking in scientific language. Academia is the practice of finding ways to break down the universe into pieces and then naming those pieces. As an academic discipline, anatomy is no exception: to this end, it makes use of the knife and Latin. Latin nomenclature affords anatomy a peculiar air of elitism as it tends to make things sound a bit more important than they actually are. To say "two heads attaches to the crow's beak" sounds sophomoric; to say "biceps attaches to the coracoid process" is scholarly.

Don't be fooled.

---

5 Of course, Bourgery's *Atlas of Human and Anatomy and Surgery* stands as a beautiful example of the perpetuation of the Humanist aesthetic into the 19th century.

The Greeks, who were responsible for the majority of ancient anatomic knowledge, did not have a classical language equivalent to our Latin with which to aggrandize their discoveries; they simply named structures after the things they resembled. For example, the small bone covering the knee resembled a saucer, and so it became the patella; the great arched vessel in the chest resembled the sheath of a sword, and so was named aorta; the smaller of the bones in the leg resembled the clasp of a toga, and was named fibula. For the ancients, naming anatomic structures was a matter of seeing the universe for what it was—it was a matter of perspective.

It is ironic that Latin became the lingua franca of anatomy. As Singer writes, despite the brutality of the Romans and their general disregard for human life, anatomic dissection was almost unknown to them; and any medical instruction that did exist in Rome would have been conducted in Greek.[6] In fact, most present day anatomic terms are simply Latinized Greek.

In this book, I have provided both English and Latin terms along with the etymology of most words. My objective in doing this is to take away the pedantic mystique of Latin—the anatomic lingo—and help students see the body the way the ancients would have: as a thing that was both a part and a reflection of the universe; a place where god—in a non-ecclesiastical sense—lies hid.[7]

I often wonder: What if the ancient Greeks had CT scans? Would they have seen them the same way they did the night sky, as constellations? Perhaps it would have gone something like this:

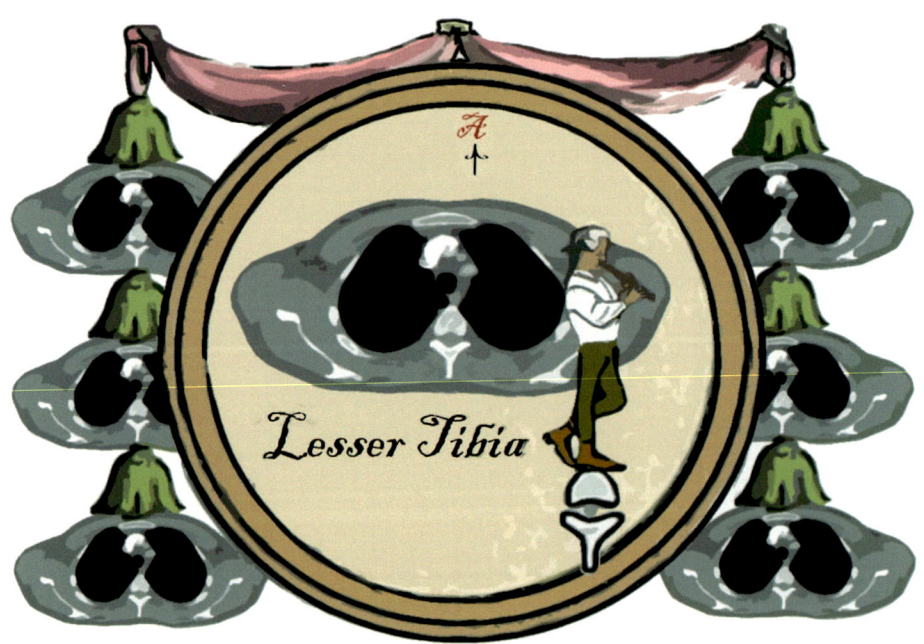

---

6 Singer, *A Short History of Anatomy and Physiology from the Greeks to Harvey.* p. 38.

7 By non-ecclesiastical, I simply mean god in a metaphorical sense and not pertaining to any specific religious doctrine. As it is well beyond the scope of this book to elaborate on any kind of theology, it is up to readers to decide for themselves what this means.

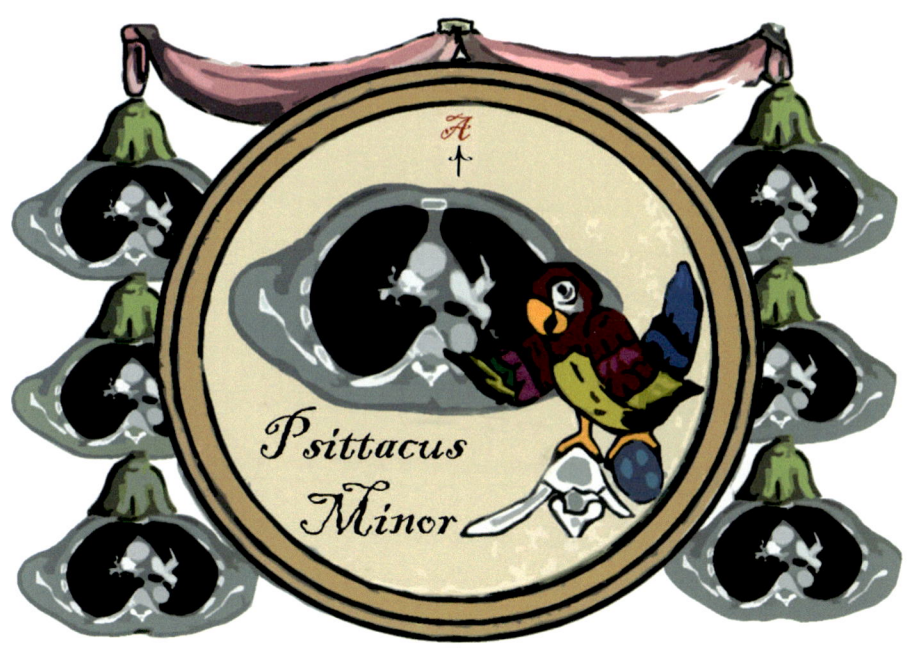

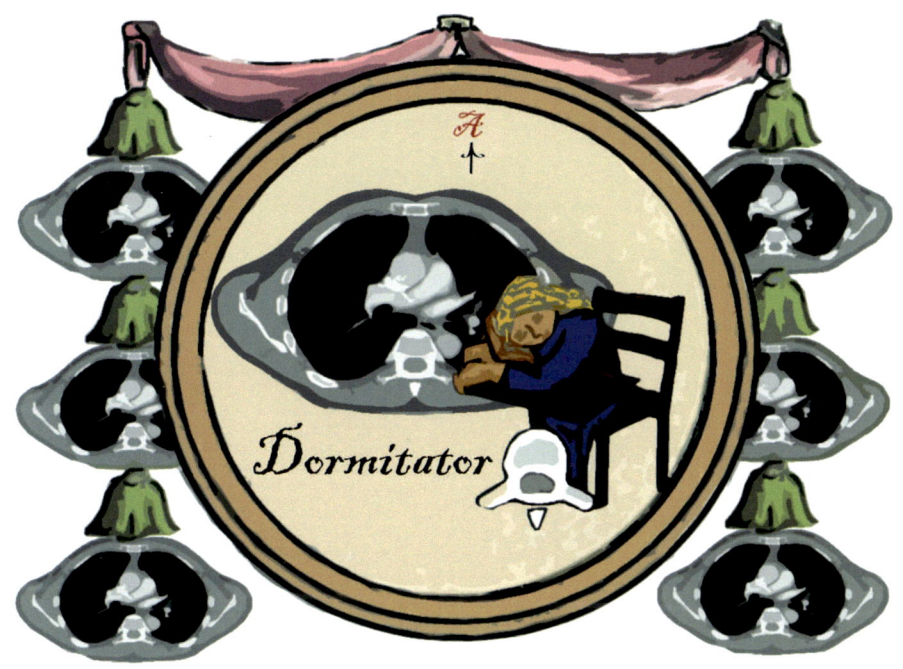

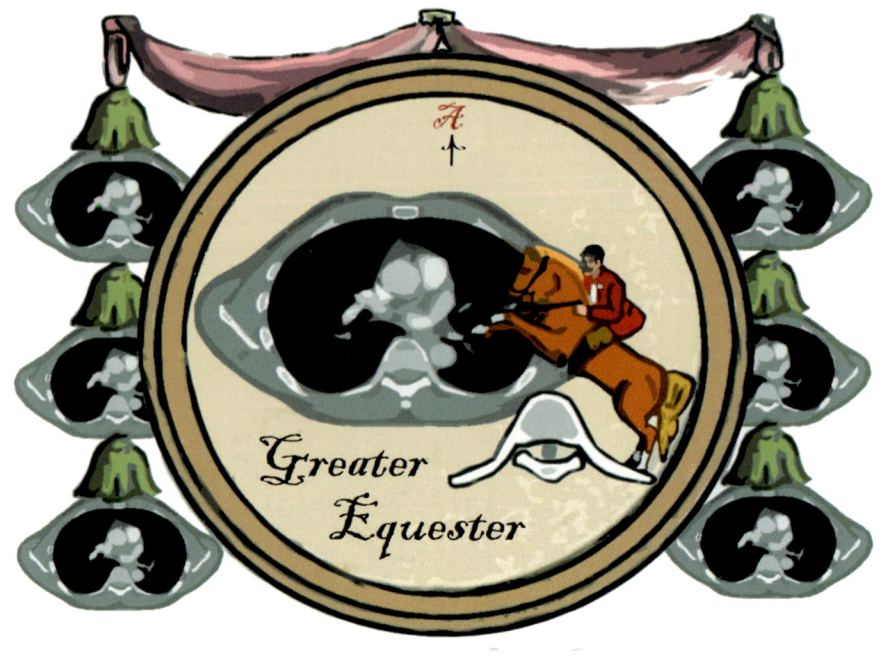

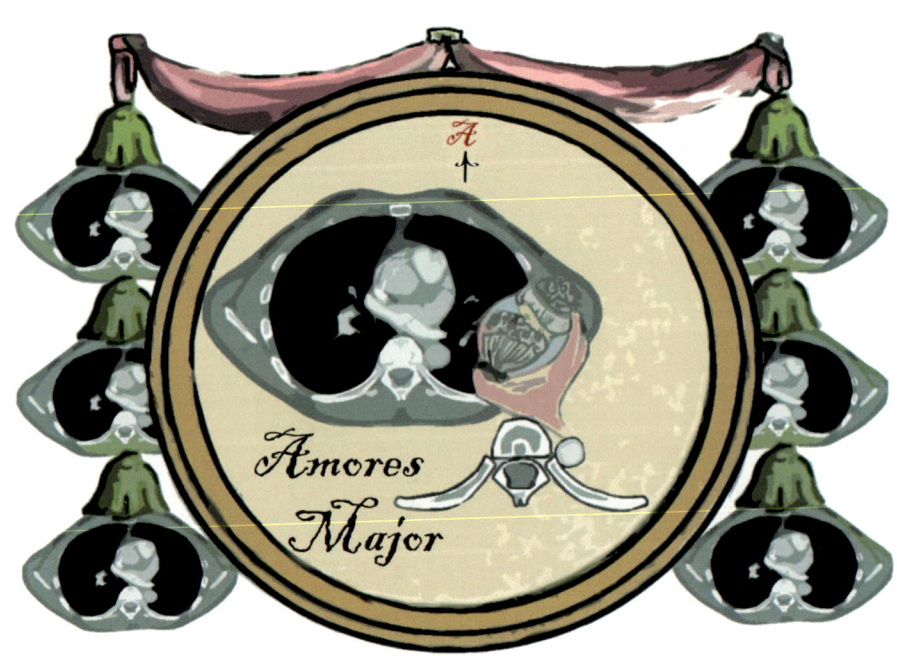

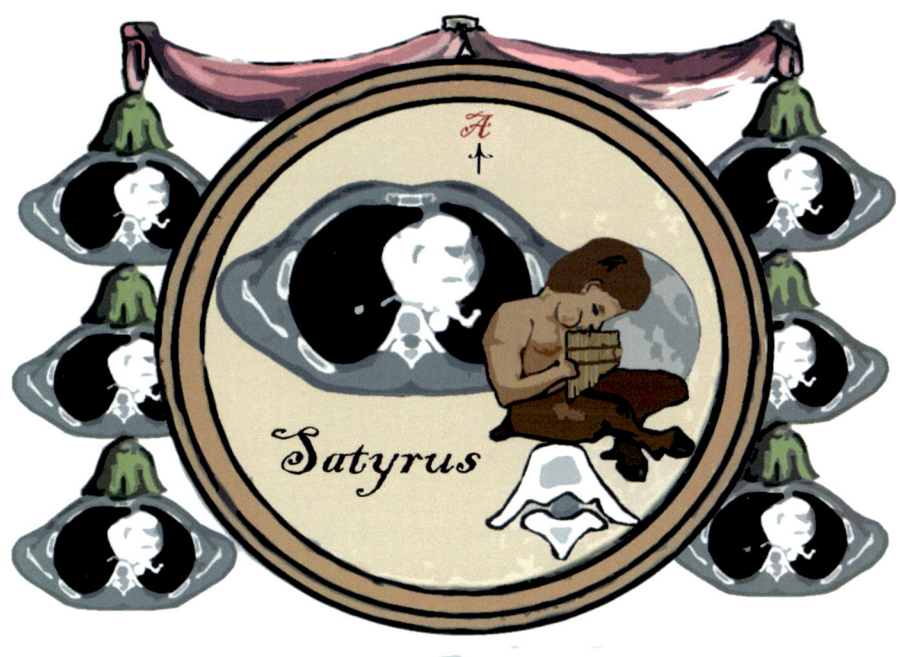

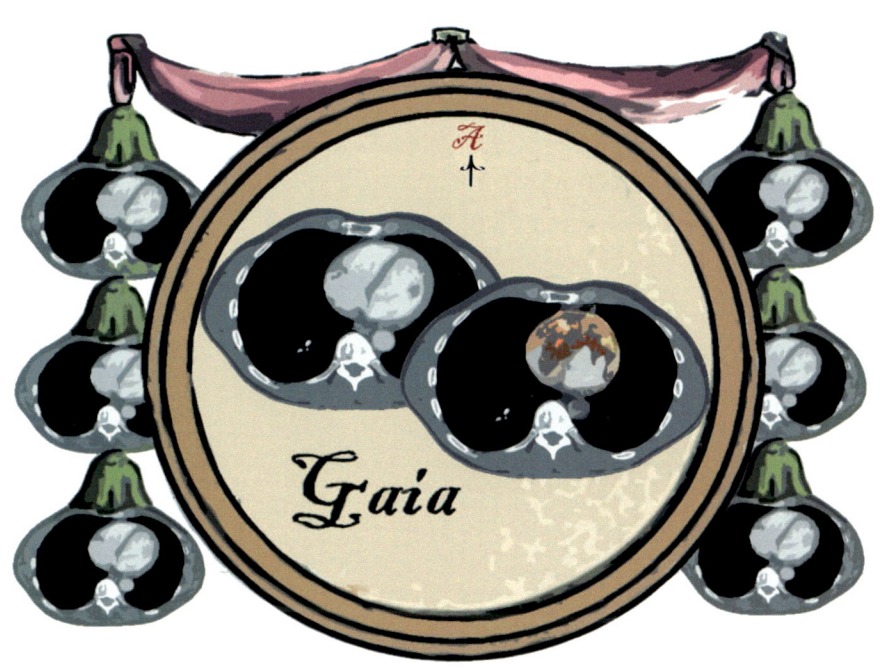

The heart, like a constellation, is a matter of perspective. It is just as arbitrary to cordon off a part of the infinite universe and call it "coronary artery" as it is to call another "Ursa Major." Boundaries, and the names applied to the things within those boundaries, are often a question of linguistics and what paradigms happen to prevail at a given time. Where the Greeks may have seen a satyr a radiologist may see the root of the great vessels. Either is as reasonable as it is capricious.[8]

These days, anatomy is considered a science. Years ago, it was where science and religion met in a peaceful union to become something else entirely. Is there a more lovely and just place for this to happen than where man's skin is peeled away? From the perspective of science, a man is composed of an infinite number of finite things; from that of religion, there is only the infinite. In flesh, where these perspectives meet, man is everything and nothing—the knower is what is known, and what is known is the knower, kissing and cutting his own warm live hand.

DJJ

Methods

This book is based on the dataset from the NIH's Visible Human Project.™[9] 3-Dimensional anatomic models were constructed using a variety of resources, including Osirix™ and Vitrea II™ imaging software. A wonderful JAVA applet, "The Visible Human Server," was also used. This latter program was developed by the École Polytechnique Fédérale de Lausanne, Computer Science Department, Peripheral Lab Systems, and is freely available on their website. Models were also created by stacking cross-sections sequentially and simply drawing in structures. These models were then used to sketch something more elaborate.

Although the anatomic illustrations are based on the Visible Human dataset, artistic license was taken in certain places. For example, the Visible Man was sectioned and imaged with his arms folded across his torso. In order to recreate the arms-above-the-head position of patients receiving a CT scan, the brachial structures seen in the cadaveric cross-sections and CT scans were removed from the cuts in Chapter 2. Further, several of the radiographic images used in the upper extremity were reconstructed and illustrated by hand. This was due to the poor quality of the available radiographic scans, again the result of the oblique angle at which the Visible Man's arms were imaged. In the pelvis chapter, the cadaver's missing testicle was reconstructed in order to create a more universal anatomy. In the thorax chapter, the central tendon of the diaphragm was illustrated in the sections showing the female breast.

Countless projects have used the Visible Human dataset in a variety of different media. These works are all available on the NIH Visible Human Project™ website. The decision of which sections to include in this work was based on what was determined to be most anatomically and clinically significant for students to learn. In 2000, The Visible Human dataset was beautifully mapped out in Dean and Herbner's "Cross-Sectional Human Anatomy." Many of the sections included by these authors were also selected for inclusion in this work.

The question of which structures to label was handled by including those deemed important for the conceptual mastery of the section. All of the English and Latin terminology used in this work is the agreed upon international anatomical terminology as published in the Federative Committee on Anatomic

---

8 One can only imagine the state of the night sky if the radiologists had gotten to it before the poets.
9 This book covers non-pathological human anatomy—illustrating human pathology in the aesthetic of this book may be a valuable contribution.

Terminology's *Terminologia Anatomica*. Greek terms and word etymologies are based on those in Henry Alan Skinner's monumental "The Origin of Medical Terms." Charles Singer's "A Short History of Anatomy and Physiology from the Greeks to Harvey" and "The Strange History of Some Anatomic Terms" was also referenced.

Several well-known and less-well known works of art are referenced throughout this book. The backgrounds from Chapter 1 are an adapted and modified version of the New York State Office of Parks, Recreation & Historic Preservation – Taconic Region's *Aqueduct Mural* which is itself adapted from *A Walker's Guide to the Old Croton Aqueduct*. These images are courtesy of New York State Office of Parks, Recreation and Historic Preservation. The backgrounds for sections I and III in chapter 3 are based on old photographs of the Village of Hastings-on-Hudson, New York, and are courtesy of the Hastings-on-Hudson Historical Society. The frontispiece preceding Chapter 1 references Michelangelo's *Separation of Light from Darkness* and William Blake's *Ancient of Days*. The frontispiece preceding Chapter 2 references a line drawing of the heart adapted from Jacopo Berengario da Carpi's *Isagogae breues, perlucidae ac uberrimae, in anatomiam humani corporis,* and is courtesy of the National Library of Medicine. The frontispiece preceding Chapter 4 references the apse of the Chapel of Fuentidueña housed at the Cloisters in Manhattan.

The figures and faces in this book were inspired from an amalgam of old tobacco cards, daguerreotypes, classical paintings, postage stamps, and people, both real and imaginary. The hairstyle of the young lady in Chapter 4 is modeled after Cyndi Lauper. The smirk on the rococo gentleman in Chapter 2 is after that in Haussmann's portrait of J. S. Bach. The moustache on the gentleman in Chapter 3 is after that of William Howard Taft. The fellow in the top hat is inspired from a 19th century tobacco card. I could not help but imagine modeling in anatomic position. As the subject of this book is the human being, its characters do what people do. They read books, wear top-hats, have piercings, smoke cigarettes, and lounge around naked—consider it either flagrant old boy'ery or just the extreme form of the four or five most commonly encountered personality types.

Finally, the judicious use of religious language and symbolism throughout this work should not be construed as proselytizing. To those intent on interpreting otherwise, please allow my use of Christian iconography to be as much an endorsement of Catholicism as my reference to satyrs is of neo-paganism.

How to Use This Book for Study

This book emphasizes conceptual mastery—not memorization. Many of the diagrams are anatomically simplified, and illustrate only those structures necessary for grasping the big picture.

Study the illustrations. Flip through the book between harder study sessions or when dining. At first, do not focus on trying to retain the minutiae. Rather, try to appreciate why things look the way they do either in an isolated section or as part of a sequence. Things will fall into place. Soon, you will begin to think multi-dimensionally.

Acknowledgments

I am greatly indebted to the authors and creators of the works referenced in this book. I would also like to acknowledge Elaine Cheung, an artist and visionary of enormous talent. Most important, this book would not have been possible in its present form without the lady and gentleman—the Visible Man and Woman— who donated themselves to better man's understanding of himself and the cosmos.

References and Works Cited

1. Balthasar, Hans Urs von. *The Glory of the Lord, Volume IV: The Realm of Metaphysics in Antiquity.* San Francisco: Ignatius Press, 1989.

2. Barleaus, Caspar. *On the place for anatomies which has recently been constructed at Amsterdam.* Schupbach, W. *The Paradox of Rembrandt's Anatomy Lesson of Dr. Nicolaes Tulp.* Med Hist Suppl. 1982; (2): 1–110.

3. Barthes, Roland. *Mythologies.* New York: Hill and Wang, 1972.

4. Berengario da Carpi, Jacopo. *Isagogae breues, perlucidae ac uberrimae, in anatomiam humani corporis.* Leaf 32. http://www.nlm.nih.gov/exhibition/historicalanatomies/home.html

5. Bougery, JM and Jacob, NH. *Atlas of Anatomy.* Los Angeles: Taschen, 2006.

6. Dean, David and Herbener, Thomas. *Cross-Sectional Human Anatomy.* New York: Lippincott, Williams, and Wilkins, 2000.

7. Federative Committee on Anatomical Terminology. *Terminologia Anatomica.* Stuttgart: Thieme, 1998.

8. Gilbert, Linda C. *A Walker's Guide to the Old Croton Aqueduct.* New York: New York State Office of Parks, Recreation & Historic Preservation and the Lucius Littauer Foundation, 1975.

9. NIH Visible Human Project™ website: http://www.nlm.nih.gov/research/visible/visible_human.html

10. Owen, Wilfred. *Maundy Thursday.* The Penguin Book of English Verse. The Penguin Group. London, England, 2004.

11. Singer, Charles. *A Short History of Anatomy and Physiology from the Greeks to Harvey.* New York: Dover, 1957.

12. Singer, Charles. *The Strange History of Some Anatomical Terms.* Med Hist. 1959 January; 3(1): 1–7.
    13. Skinner, Henry Alan. *The Origin of Medical Terms.* New York: Hafner Pub. Co., 1970.

14. Vesalius, Andreas. *De corporis humani fabrica libri septem.* http://www.nlm.nih.gov/exhibition/historicalanatomies/home.html

Figure Legend

From Andreas Vesalius' *De corporis humani fabrica libri septem.* Courtesy of the National Library of Medicine.

CHAPTER ONE
THE HEAD AND NECK

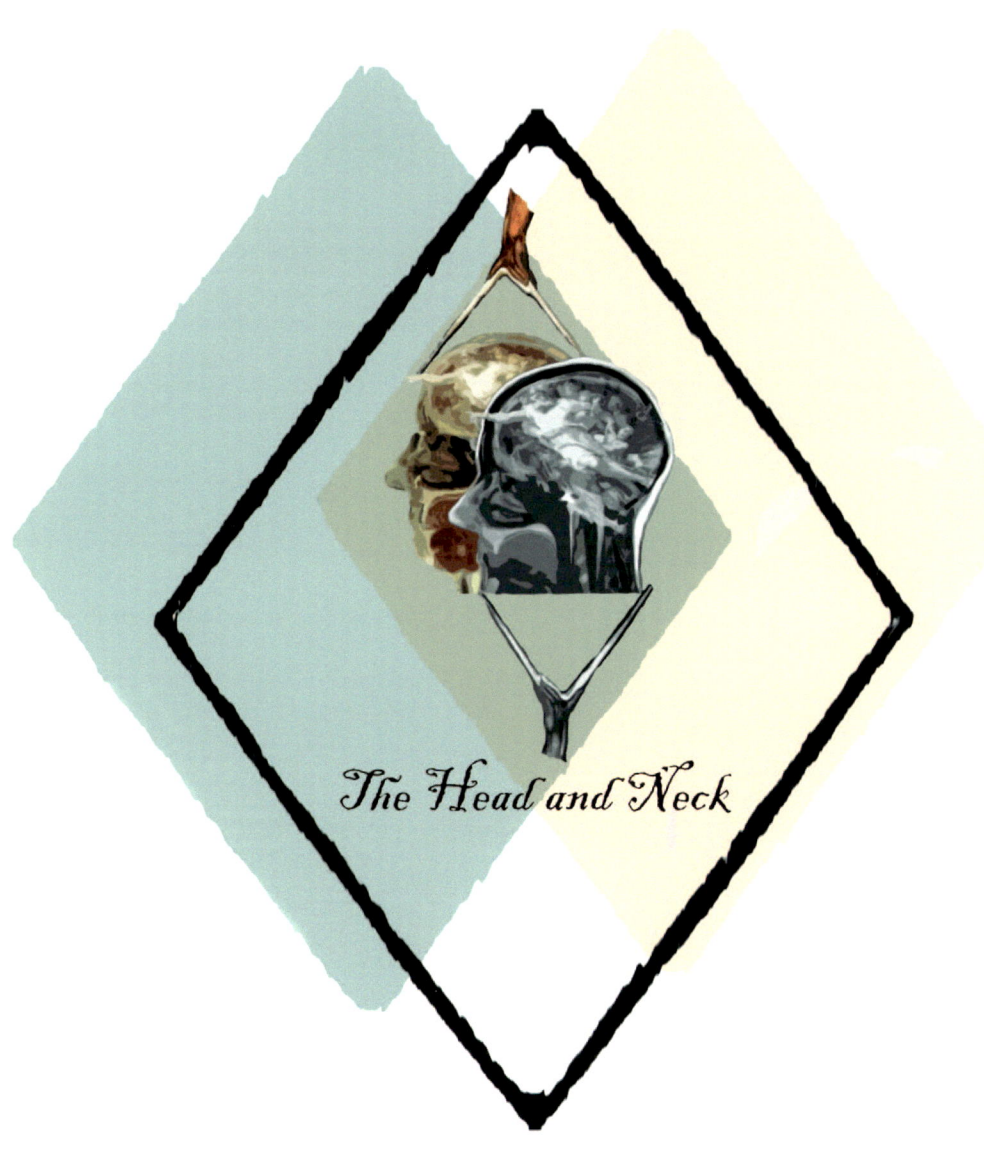

The Head and Neck

Part One:
The Head

1 – Superior Cranium and the Frontal Sinus

The head has been sliced slightly inferior to the most superior aspect of the skull. This section demonstrates the relation of the frontal sinus to its over and underlying structures. The frontal sinus, the hollow space in the frontal bone that drains into the nasal cavity, is lined with a mucoperiosteum. It is significant in several pathological processes, from sinus infections to head traumas. Note the relation of the brain to the posterior plate of the frontal sinus. When this structure is fractured the brain is threatened with infection, as it is exposed to the external environment through the nasal cavity. The sinus may be further appreciated in the corresponding CT scan.

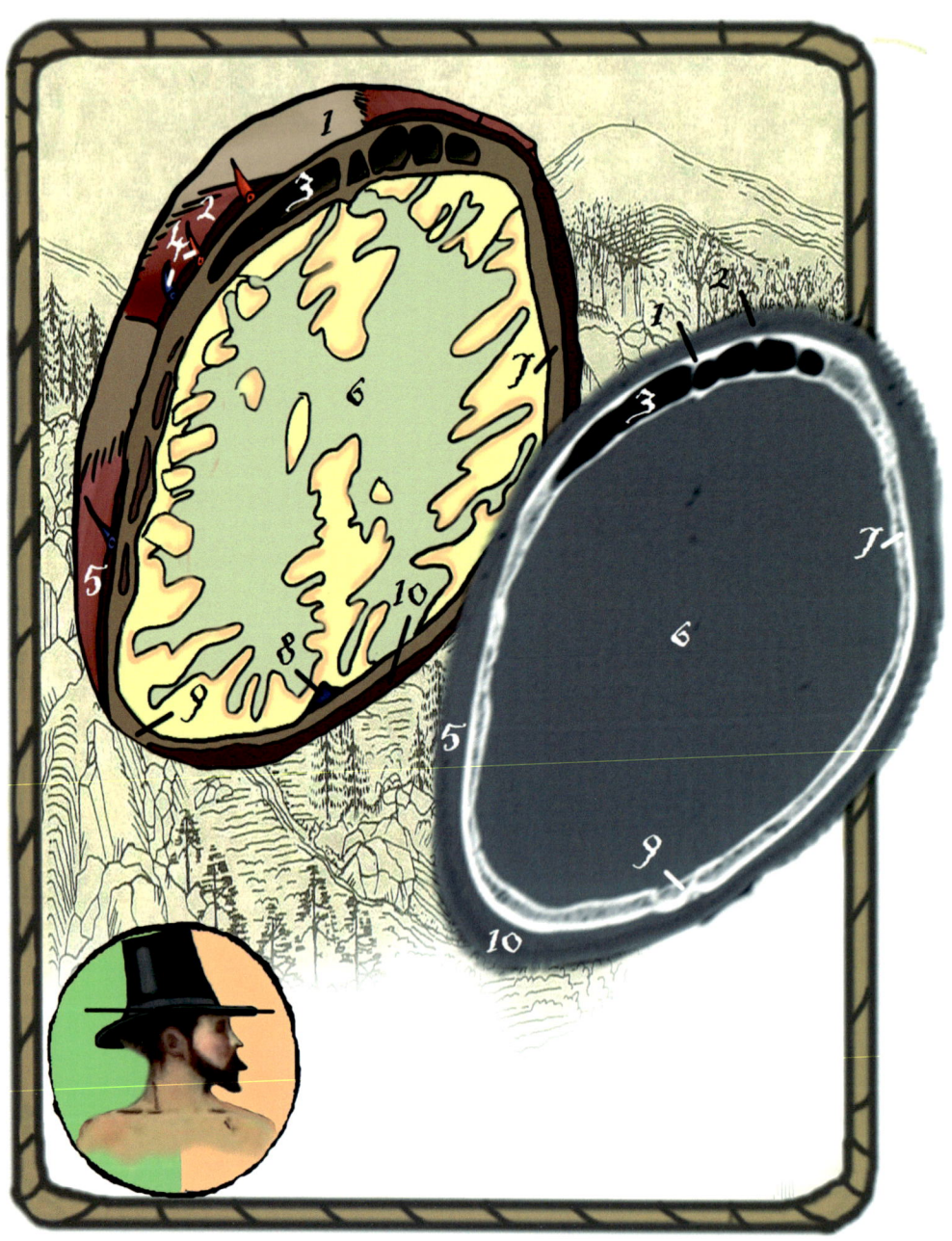

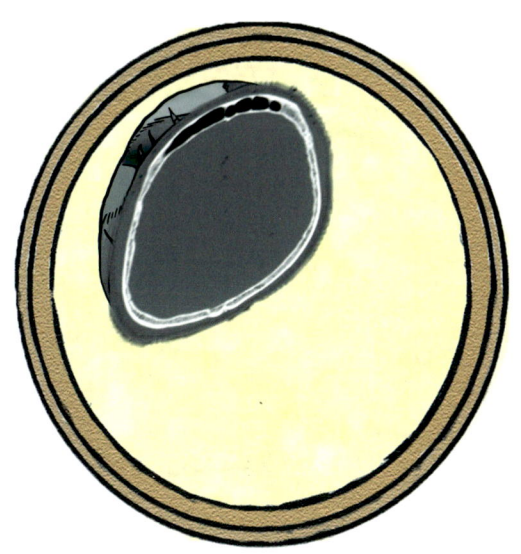

8. **Superior sagittal sinus** (*Sinus sagittalis superior*) Sagittal, from the Latin, sagittal, meaning arrow. Sagittarius is an archer. The term was likely applied to the head for the resemblance of the sagittal suture to an arrow.

9. **Occipital bone** (*Os occipitale*) A combination of the Latin terms ob, meaning opposite, or against, and caput, meaning head. Occipitus is the back of the head.

10. **Occipital belly of occipitofrontalis** (*M. occipitofrontalis, venter occipitalis*)

1. **Frontal bone** (*Os frontal*)

2. **Frontal belly of occipitofrontalis** (*M. occipitofrontalis, venter frontalis*)

3. **Frontal sinus** (*Sinus frontalis*)

4. **Superficial temporal artery and vein** (*Arteria et vena temporalis superficialis*)

5. **Temporalis** (*M. temporalis*)

6. **Cerebrum** (*Cerebrum*) Named by Eristratus of Alexandria in the 3rd century BC, the term is derived from the Latin word for brain.

7. **Parietal bone** (*Os parietale*) Derived from the Latin term for wall, paries.

II – The Mid-Orbit

In this section the head has been sliced through the middle of the oculus. The structures of the orbital socket can be appreciated, and the relation of the oculus to the adjacent nasal bone. The nasal bone sits at 12 o'clock, its septum seen in the midline. Medial and lateral rectus can be seen in cross section on either side of the oculus. A wisp of superior rectus can be appreciated behind the right optic nerve. The optic nerves can be followed to the optic chiasm and to the cruciate optic tract. Note the proximity of the cerebrum to the ethmoid air cells and the sphenoid sinus. The temporal fat pad has been removed on the left side in order to allow the underlying temporalis muscle to be better visualized. Many of these same structures can be seen in the corresponding CT.

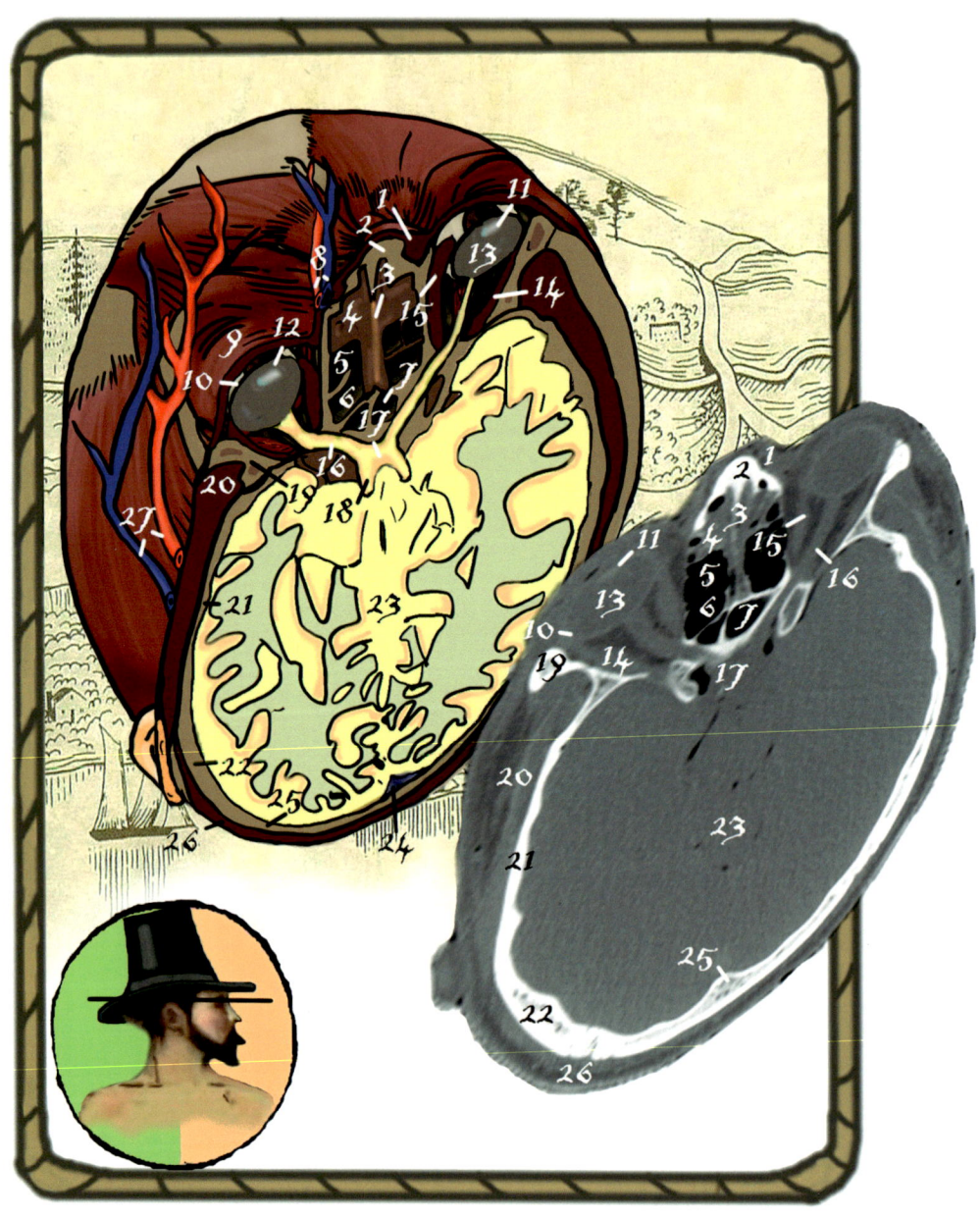

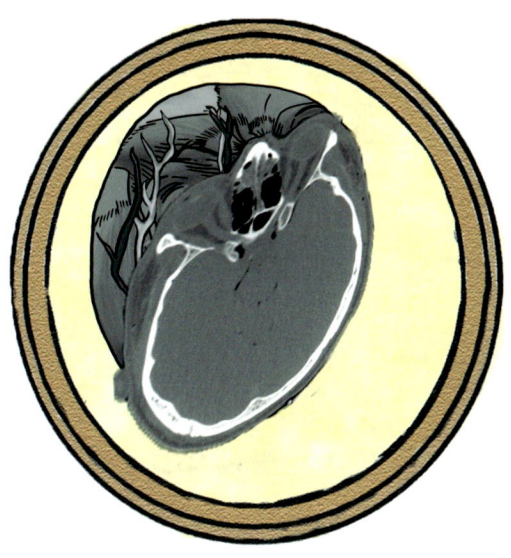

1. **Procerus muscle** (*M. procerus*)

2. **Nasal bone** (*Os nasale*)

3. **Nasal septum** (*Septum nasi*)

4. **Anterior ethmoid cells** (*Cellulae ethmoidales anteriores*) Derived from ηθμος, meaning a sieve, the ethmoid bone was named by Galen.

5. **Middle ethmoid cells** (*Os ethmoidale, cellulae ethmoidales mediae*)

6. **Posterior ethmoid cells** (*Os ethmoidale, cellulae ethmoidales posteriores*)

7. **Sphenoid sinus** (*Sinus sphenoidalis*)

8. **Supraorbital artery and vein** (Arteria et vena supraorbitalis)

9. **Obicularis oculi** (*M. obicularis oculi*) From the Latin orbiculus, meaning a small disc, the muscle was named by Douglas in the 18th century.

10. **Oculus** (*Bulbus oculi*)

11. **Lens** (*Lens*)

12. **Anterior chamber** (*Camera anterior*)

13. **Posterior chamber** (*Camera posterior*)

14. **Lateral rectus** (*M. rectus lateralis*)

15. **Medial rectus** (*M. rectus medialis*)

16. **Optic nerve** (*Nervus opticus*)

17. **Optic chiasm** (*Chiasma opticum*)

18. **Optic tract** (*Tractus opticus*)

19. **Greater wing of the sphenoid bone** (*Os sphenoidale, ala major*) Derived from σφηνοειδης, meaning wedge-shaped, the bone was named by Galen.

20. **Temporalis** (*M. temporalis*)

21. **Temporal bone** (*Os temporale*)

22. **Parietal bone** (*Os parietale*)

23. **Cerebrum** (*Cerebrum*)

24. **Superior sagittal sinus** (*Sinus sagittalis superior*)

25. **Occipital bone** (*Os occipitale*)

26. **Occipital belly of occipitofrontalis** (*M. occipitofrontalis, venter occipitalis*)

27. **Superficial temporal artery and vein** (*Arteria et vena temporalis superficialis*)

III – The Inferior Orbit and Sphenoid Sinus

In this section, the head has been sliced through the inferior aspect of the orbit. The nasal septum sits at 12 o'clock, and the ethmoid air cells are seen on either side. Inferior oblique is seen in cross section beneath either eye, as well as inferior rectus. Beneath the eyes, the hollow cavity of the maxillary sinus can be seen for the first time, while the sphenoid sinus occupies a position in the midline. Directly posterior to the sphenoid sinus sits the pons. Lateral to the sphenoid sinus, the cavernous sinus is seen, with the internal carotid artery running its course therein. Notice that the temporal fat pad has been removed from the left in order to better visualize temporalis. Many of these structures have been captured in the corresponding CT scan.

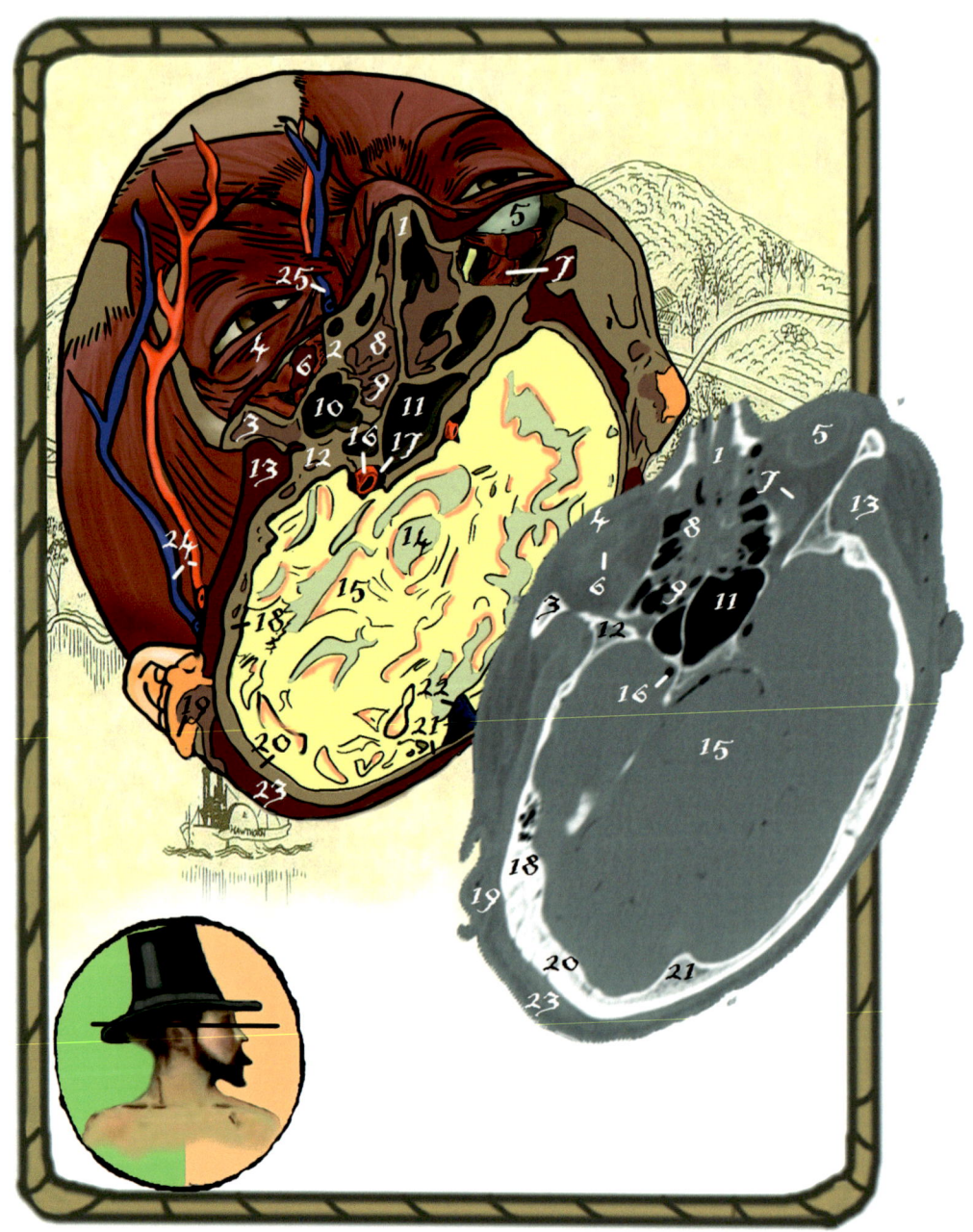

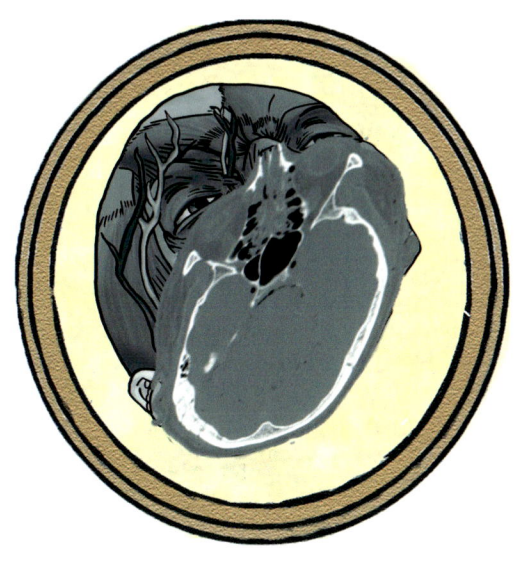

1. **Nasal septum** (*Septum nasi*)

2. **Frontal process of the maxilla** (*Maxilla, processus frontalis*) Derived from mala, meaning cheek, the bone was named by Celsus in the 1st century.

3. **Frontal process of the zygomatic bone** (*Os zygomaticum, processus frontalis*) Derived from ζυγόμα, meaning yoke, the device used to harness farm animals, the bone was named by Galen

4. **Obicularis oculi** (*M. obicularis oculi*)

5. **Oculus** (*Bulbus oculi*)

6. **Inferior oblique** (*M. obliquus inferior*)

7. **Inferior rectus** (*M. rectus inferior*)

8. **Middle ethmoid cells** (*Os ethmoidale, cellulae ethmoidales mediae*)

9. **Posterior ethmoid cells** (*Os ethmoidale, cellulae ethmoidales posteriores*)

10. **Maxillary sinus** (*Sinus maxillaris*)

11. **Sphenoid sinus** (*Sinus sphenoidalis*)

12. **Greater wing of the sphenoid bone** (*Os sphenoidale, ala major*)

13. **Temporalis** (*M. temporalis*)

14. **Pons** (*Pons*)

15. **Cerebrum** (*Cerebrum*)

16. **Internal carotid artery** (*Arteria carotis interna*) Carotid is derived from καρωτίδα, meaning to make sleepy, as the ancients noted this effect in animals when pressure was applied to the vessel in the neck.

17. **Cavernous sinus** (*Sinus cavernosus*)

18. **Temporal bone** (*Os temporale*)

19. **Auricular cartilage** (*Cartilago auriculae*)

20. **Parietal bone** (*Os parietale*)

21. **Occipital bone** (*Os occipitale*)

22. **Superior sagittal sinus** (*Sinus sagittalis superior*)

23. **Occipital belly of occipitofrontalis** (*M. occipitofrontalis, venter occipitalis*)

24. **Superficial temporal artery and vein** (*Arteria et vena temporalis superficialis*)

25. **Angular vein** (*V. angularis*)

IV – The Maxillary Sinus

The head has been sliced through the middle of the bridge of the nose and the mid-point of the maxillary bone. The nasal septum occupies the 12 o'clock position, and on either side, the hollow cavities of the maxillary sinuses are quite prominent. The acoustic meatus can be seen at the 3 o'clock position. Masseter is seen for the first time, and near the arising mandible, lateral pterygoid and temporalis make an appearance. The cerebellum sits posteriorly. Many of these structures may be appreciated in the corresponding CT.

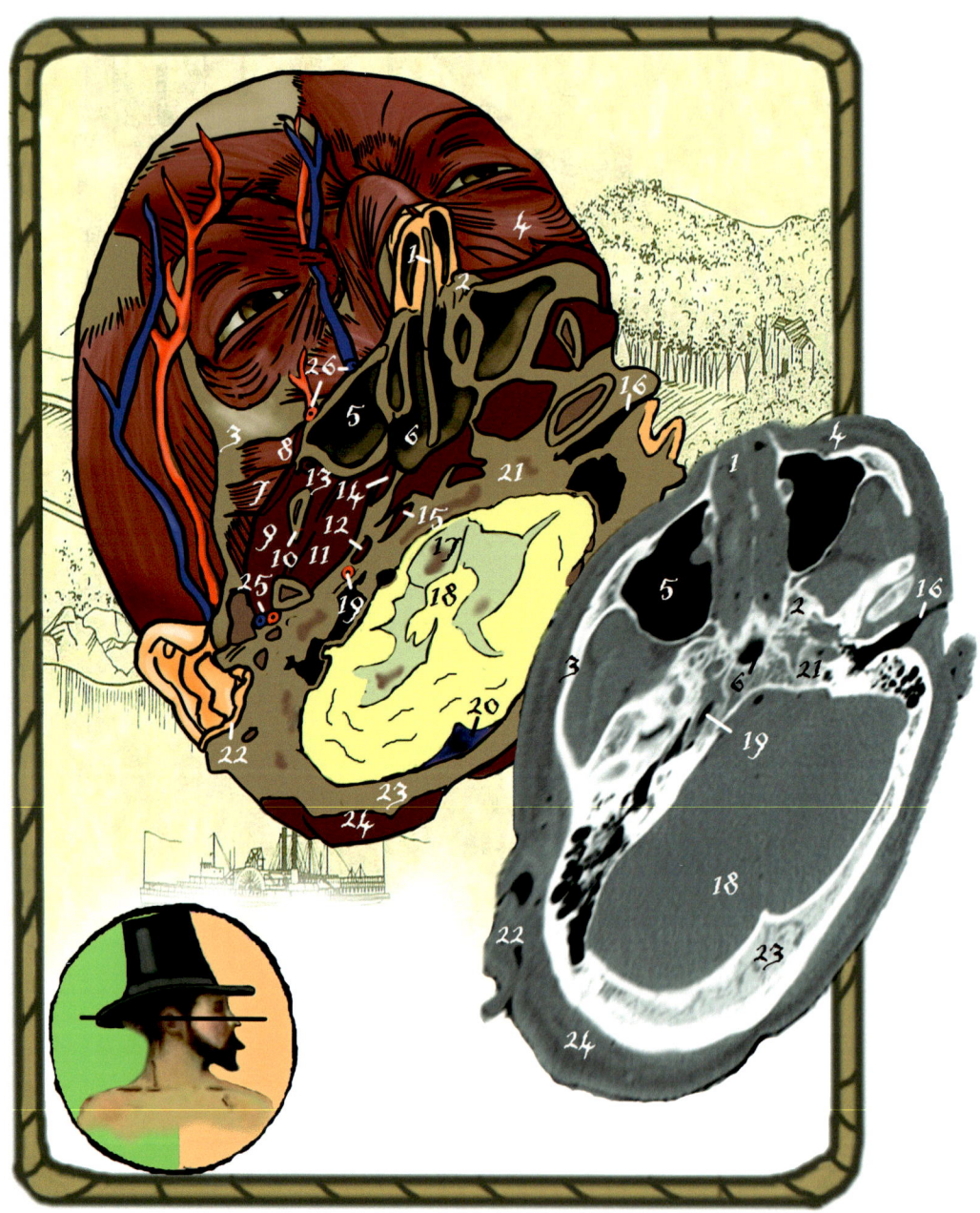

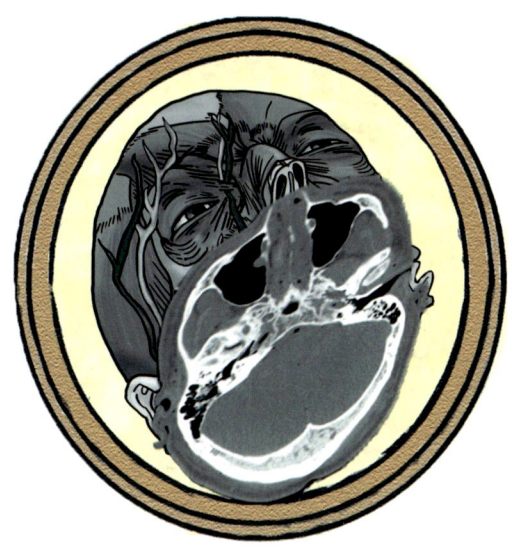

1. **Nasal septum** (*Septum nasi*)

2. **Frontal process of the maxilla** (*Maxilla, processus frontalis*)

3. **Zygomatic bone** (*Os zygomaticum*)

4. **Obicularis oculi** (*M. obicularis oculi*)

5. **Maxillary sinus** (*Sinus maxillaris*)

6. **Sphenoid sinus** (*Sinus sphenoidalis*)

7. **Zygomaticus major** (*M. zygomaticus major*)

8. **Zygomaticus minor** (*M. zygomaticus minor*)

9. **Masseter** (*M. masseter*) Derived from μασητήρ, meaning chewer, the muscle was named by Galen.

10. **Mandible** (*Mandibula*)

11. **Lateral pterygoid** (*M. pterygoideus lateralis*) Derived πτερυζ, meaning a wing, the muscles were named by Riolan in the 17th century.

12. **Tensor veli palatini** (*M. tensor veli palatini*)

13. **Temporalis** (*M. temporalis*)

14. **Medial pterygoid** (*M. pterygoideus medialis*)

15. **Longus capitis** (*M. longus capitis*)

16. **External acoustic meatus** (*Meatus acusticus externus*)

17. **Pons** (*Pons*)

18. **Cerebellum** (*Cerebellum*) Derived from cerebrum, meaning little brain, and first used by Eristratus of Alexandria in the 3rd century BC.

19. **Internal carotid artery** (*Arteria carotis interna*)

20. **Superior sagittal sinus** (*Sinus sagittalis superior*)

21. **Temporal bone** (*Os temporale*)

22. **Auricular cartilage** (*Cartilago auriculae*)

23. **Occipital bone** (*Os occipitale*)

24. **Occipital belly of occipitofrontalis** (*M. occipitofrontalis, venter occipitalis*)

25. **Superficial temporal artery and vein** (*Arteria et vena temporalis superficialis*)

26. **Facial artery and vein** (*Arteria et vena facialis*)

V – Atlo-Axial Joint – C-1/C-2

In this section the head has been sliced through the interior aspect of the maxilla. This is level to the atlo-axial joint, which can be appreciated in posterior mid-line. Obicularis oris sits at 12 o'clock anteriorly. The arch of the maxilla, which houses the alveoli in which sit the teeth, can also be seen. The tongue and soft palate sit posterior to the maxilla. The parotid glands sit at 10 and 2 o'clock, and medial to these are masseter, the mandible, and medial pterygoid. Posteriorly, the dens of the axis is surrounded by the atlas, while the deep muscles of the head and neck surround one another like bandages. The shape of the atlo-axial joint has been captured quite well in the corresponding CT scan.

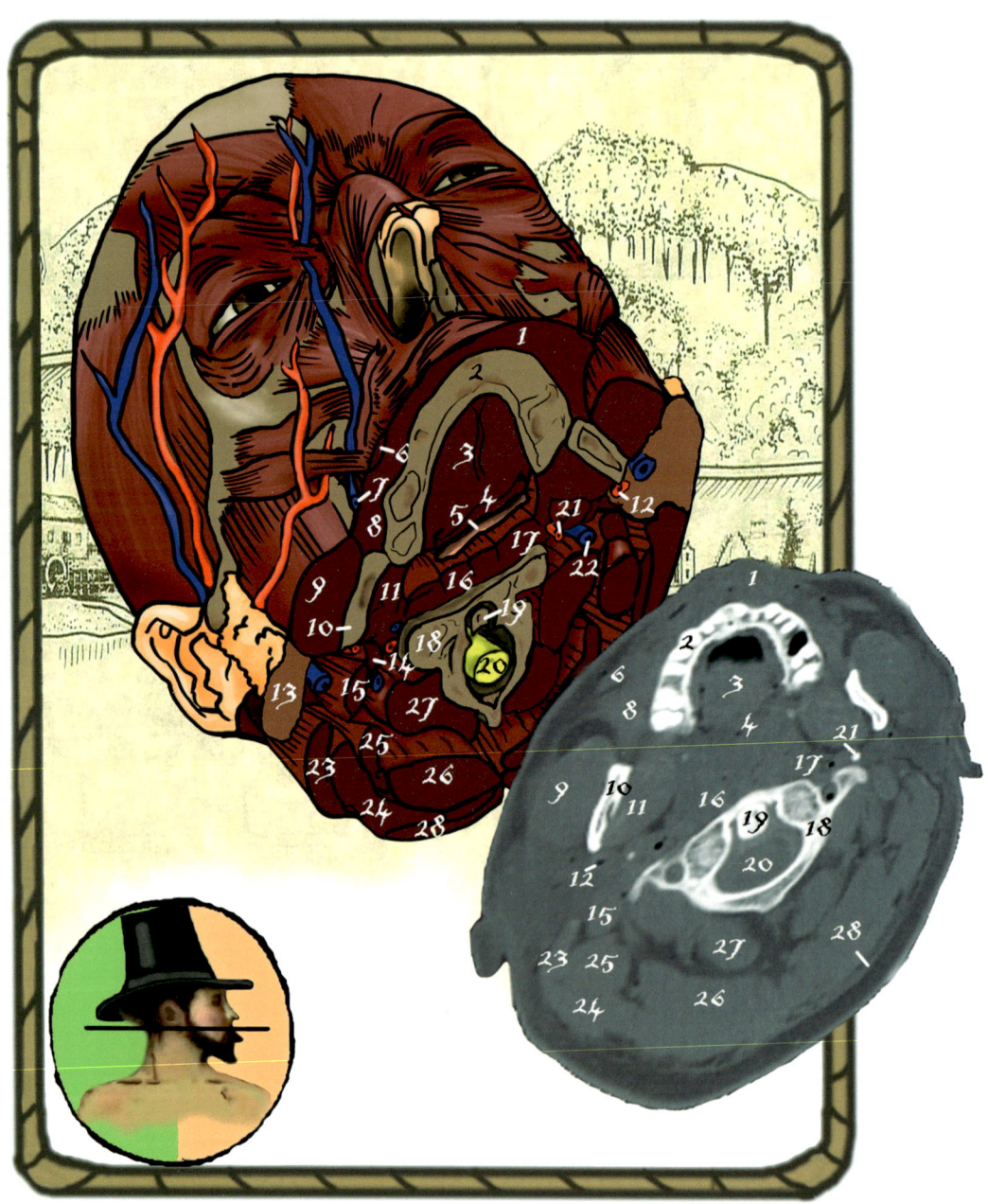

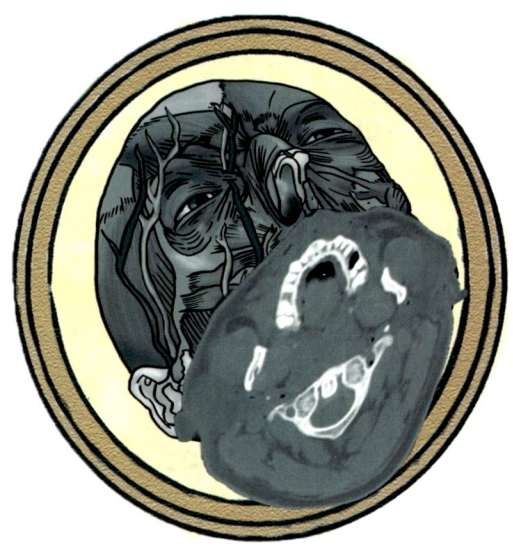

1. **Obicularis oris** (*M. obicularis oris*) Derived from the Latin terms for a small disc, and mouth, the muscle was named by Albinus in the 18th century.

2. **Maxilla** (*Os maxilla*)

3. **Tongue** (*Lingua*)

4. **Soft palate** (*Palatum molle/velle palatinum*)

5. **Pharynx** (*Pharynx*) Derived from φάρνξ, meaning throat, the term was first used by Galen.

6. **Zygomaticus major** (*M. zygomaticus major*)

7. **Facial vein** (*Vena facialis*)

8. **Buccinator** (*M. buccinator*) Derived from the Latin, bucina, meaning term for trumpeter.

9. **Masseter** (*M. masseter*)

10. **Mandible** (*Mandibula*)

11. **Medial pterygoid** (*M. pterygoideus medialis*)

12. **Retromandibular artery and vein** (*Arteria et vena retromandibularis*)

13. **Parotid gland** (*Glandula parotidea*) Derived from, παρωτίς meaning next to the ear, the term was used by Hippocrates.

14. **Stylohyoid** (*M. stylohyoideus*) Derived from στυλος, meaning a long pillar, the muscle was named by Eustachius in the 16th century, although the bony process was named by Galen.

15. **Posterior belly of the digastric** (*M. digastricus, venter posterior*) Derived from the Greek term for two bellies, the muscle was named by Galen.

16. **Longus colli** (*M. longus colli*)

17. **Longus capitis** (*M. longus capitis*)

18. **Atlas, CI** (*Atlas*) Named for Atlas, the mythological hero turned to stone by Perseus with medusa's head. The term was once applied to the 7th cervical vertebra, but was later applied to the 1st by Vesalius.

19. **Dens of C2, Axis** (*Axis*) Derived from άξων, meaning axle, the bone was named by the lexicographer Julius Pollux in the 2nd century.

20. **Spinal Cord** (*Medulla spinalis*)

21. **Internal carotid artery** (*Arteria carotis interna*)

22. **Internal jugular vein** (*Vena jugularis interna*) Named by Galen, the term is derived from jugulum, the Latin term for throat.

23. **Sternocleidomastoid** (*M. sternocleidomastoideus*)

24. **Splenius capitis** (*M. splenius capitis*) Derived from σπληνιου, meaning a bandage. The deep muscles of the head and neck were thought to wrap around each other, like bandages.

25. **Longissimus capitis** (*M. longissimus capitis*)

26. **Semispinalis capitis** (*M. semispinalis capitis*)

27. **Rectus capitis** (*M. rectus capitis*)

28. **Trapezius** (*M. trapezius*) Derived from τραπέζιου, meaning a small table, the muscle was named by Galen.

VI – Mid-Mandible – C-3

In this section, the head has been sliced through the inferior aspect of the mid-mandible. The mandible is surrounded by the facial muscles anteriorly, such as obicularis oris. Posteriorly, genioglossus straddles the midline, and at about the 10 and 2 o'clock position is mylohyoid, with hyoglossus more medial. The submandibular glands sit at about 9 and 3 o'clock, with sternocleidomastoid at 8 and 4 o'clock. Posteriorly arc the deep head and neck muscles. A corresponding CT is shown.

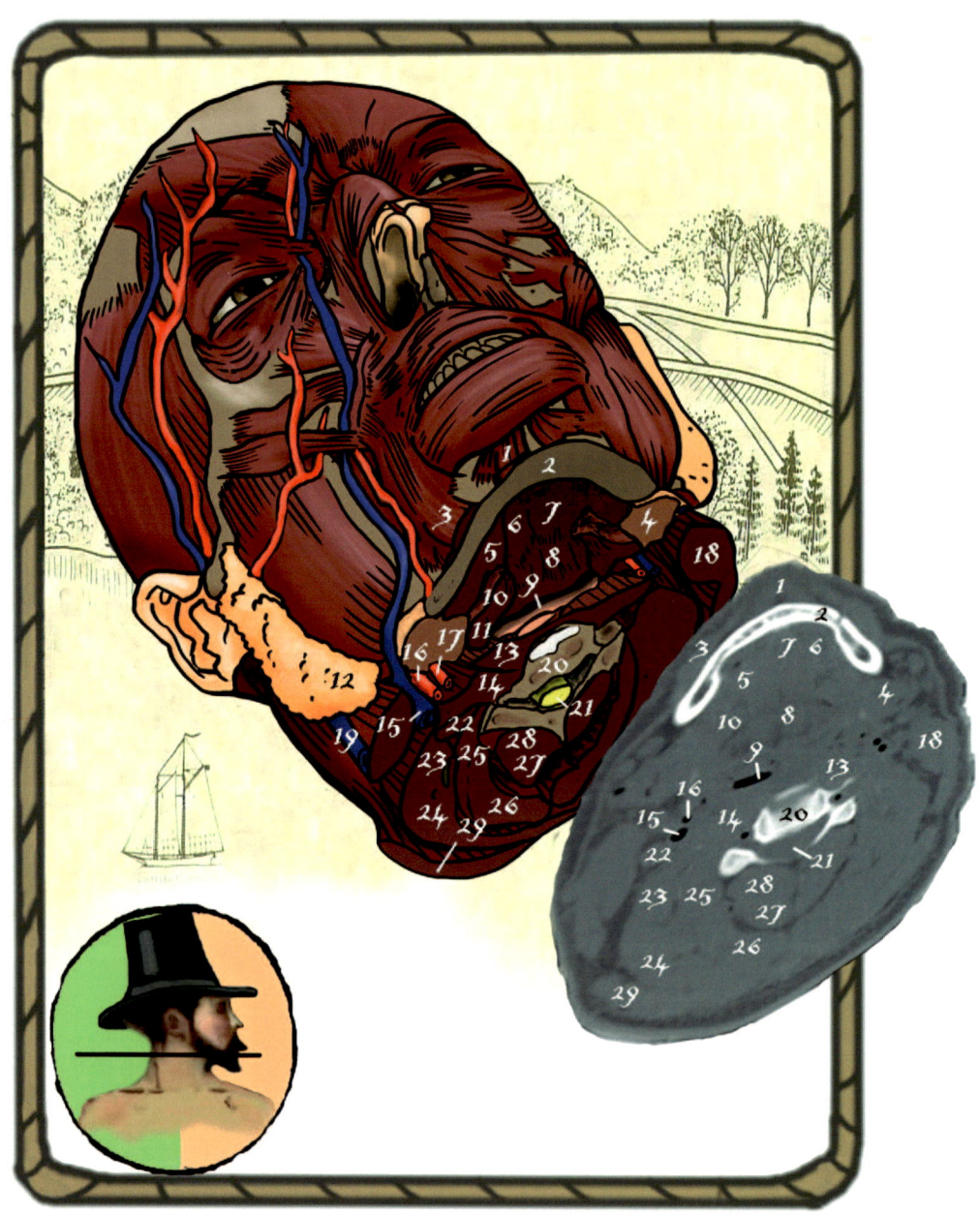

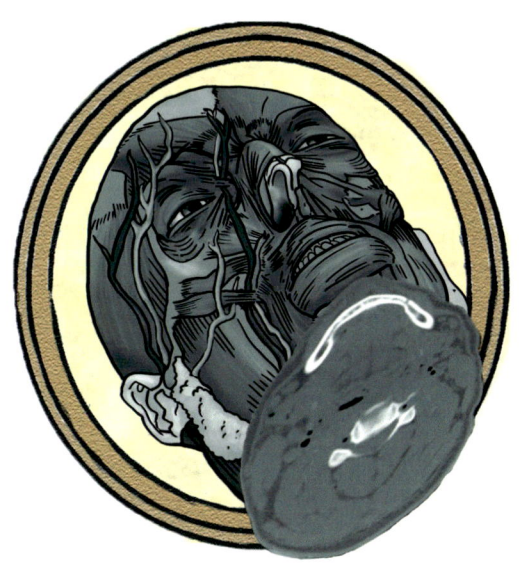

17. **Internal carotid artery** (*Arteria carotis interna*)

18. **Sternocleidomastoid** (*M. sternocleidomastoideus*)

19. **External jugular vein** (*Vena jugularis externa*)

20. **Third cervical vertebra** (*Vertebra cervicale tertia*) The term vertebra, derived from vertere, Latin for to rotate or to turn, was first used by Celsus.

21. **Spinal Cord** (*Medulla spinalis*)

22. **Posterior scalene** (*M. scalenus posterior*) Derived from σκαληνός, meaning an irregular sided triangle, the muscles were named by Riolan in the 17th century.

23. **Levator scapulae** (*M. levator scapulae*)

24. **Splenius capitis** (*M. splenius capitis*)

25. **Splenius cervicis** (*M. splenius cervicis*)

26. **Semispinalis capitis** (*M. semispinalis capitis*)

27. **Semispinalis cervicis** (*M. semispinalis cervicis*)

28. **Erector spinae** (*Musculus erector spinae*)

29. **Trapezius** (*M. trapezius*)

1. **Mentalis** (*M. mentalis*)

2. **Mandible** (*Mandibula*)

3. **Depressor anguli oris** (*M. depressor anguli oris*)

4. **Submandibular gland** (*Glandula submandibularis*)

5. **Mylohyoid** (*M. mylohyoideus*) Derived from μυλου, meaning the lower jaw, the muscle was named by Cowper in the 17th century.

6. **Geniohyoid** (*M. geniohyoideus*)

7. **Genioglossus** (*M. genioglossus*)

8. **Tongue** (*Lingua*)

9. **Pharynx** (*Pharynx*)

10. **Hyoglossus** (*M. hyoglossus*)

11. **Stylohyoid** (*M. stylohyoideus*)

12. **Parotid gland** (*Glandula parotidea*)

13. **Superior pharyngeal constrictor** (*M. constrictor pharyngis superior*)

14. **Longus colli** (*M. longus colli*)

15. **Internal jugular vein** (*Vena jugularis interna*)

16. **External carotid artery** (*Arteria carotis externa*)

VII – Inferior Mandible – C-4

The head has been sliced through the most inferior aspect of the mandible. The platysma has been removed in order to better visualize the underlying structures of the neck. The mandible sits at 12 o'clock. Three distinct muscle groups sit beneath this structure. From lateral to medial, these are the anterior belly of digastric, mylohyoid, and geniohyoid. The hyoid, a U-shaped bone, can be seen posterior to these muscles, and posterior still, the pharynx. The submandibular glands sit at 10 and 2 o'clock, while sternocleidomastoid sits at 9 and 3. Medial to sternocleidomastoid, the right common carotid artery is seen as it bifurcates into internal and external branches. In the midline is the fourth cervical vertebra. A corresponding CT shows these structures radiographically.

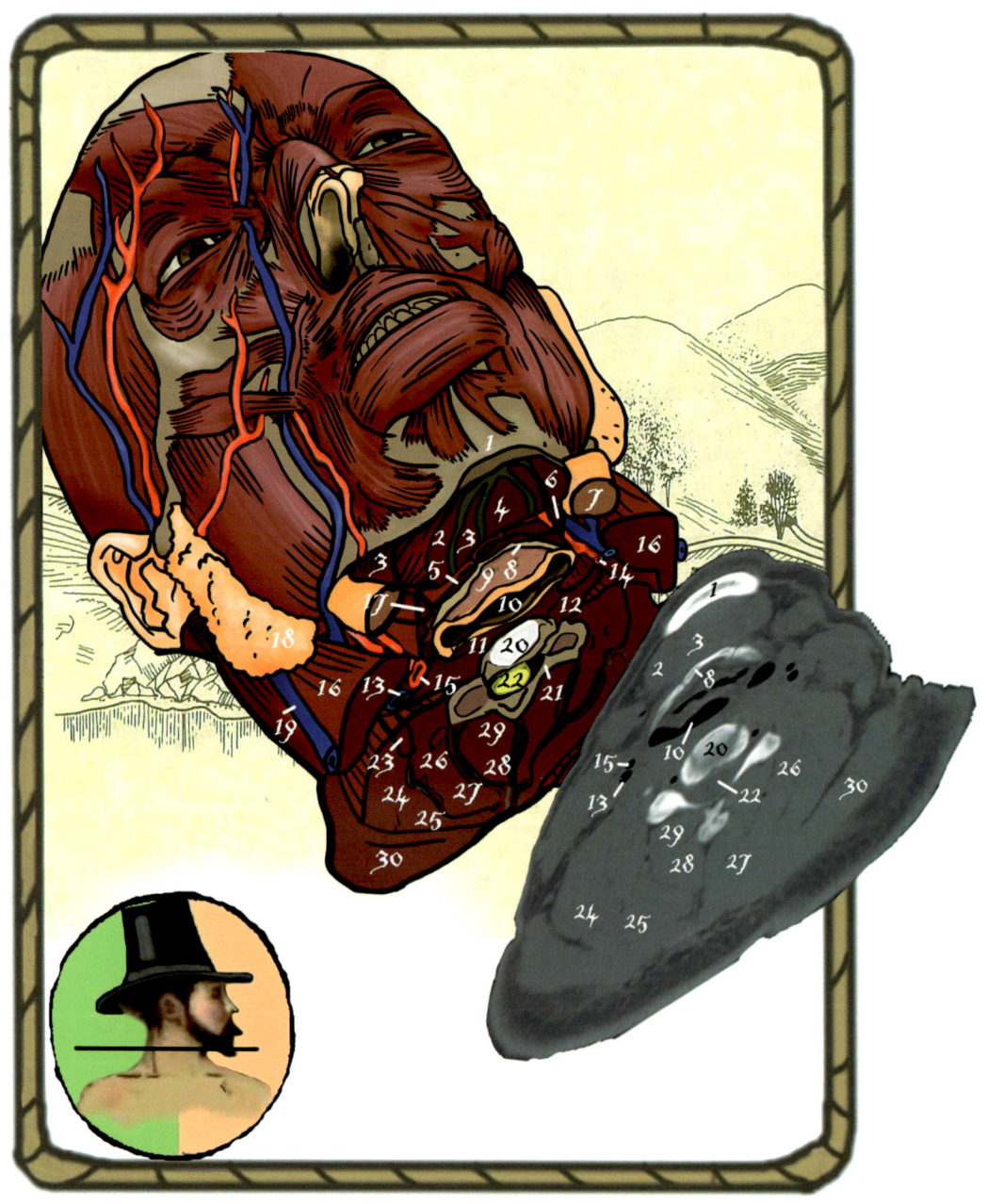

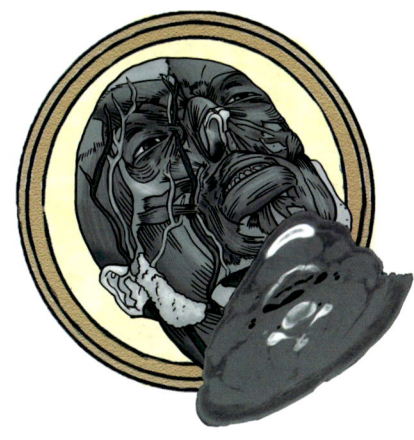

1. **Mandible** (*Mandibula*)
2. **Anterior belly of the digastric** (*M. digastricus, venter anterior*)
3. **Mylohyoid** (*M. mylohyoideus*)
4. **Geniohyoid** (*M. geniohyoideus*)
5. **Hyoglossus** (*M. hyoglossus*)
6. **Posterior belly of the digastric** (*M. digastricus, venter posterior*)
7. **Submandibular gland** (*Glandula submandibularis*)
8. **Hyoid** (*Os hyoideum*) The bone, named for the Greek letter upsilon, or U, was named by Herophilus of Alexandria in the 3rd century BC.
9. **Epiglottic vallecula** (*Vallecula epiglottica*)
10. **Pharynx** (*Pharynx*)
11. **Superior pharyngeal constrictor** (*M. constrictor pharyngis superior*)
12. **Longus colli** (*M. longus colli*)
13. **Internal jugular vein** (*Vena jugularis interna*)
14. **Internal carotid artery** (*Arteria carotis interna*)
15. **Bifurcation of the common carotid artery** (*Bifurcatio carotidis*)
16. **Sternocleidomastoid** (*M. sternocleidomastoideus*)
17. **Stylohyoid** (*M. stylohyoideus*)
18. **Parotid gland** (*Glandula parotidea*)
19. **External jugular vein** (*Vena jugularis externa*)
20. **Intervertebral disk between the third and fourth cervical vertebrae** (*Discus intervertebralis*)
21. **Fourth cervical vertebra** (*Vertebra cervicale quarta*)
22. **Spinal Cord** (*Medulla spinalis*)
23. **Posterior scalene** (*M. scalenus posterior*)
24. **Levator scapulae** (*M. levator scapulae*)
25. **Splenius capitis** (*M. splenius capitis*)
26. **Splenius cervicis** (*M. splenius cervicis*)
27. **Semispinalis capitis** (*M. semispinalis capitis*)
28. **Semispinalis cervicis** (*M. semispinalis cervicis*)
29. **Erector spinae** (*Musculus erector spinae*)
30. **Trapezius** (*M. trapezius*)

Part Two:
The Neck

VIII – The Thyroid Cartilage – C-5

In this section, the neck has been sliced slightly inferior to the chin, at the level of the thyroid cartilage. This cartilage, known colloquially as the Adam's apple, straddles the midline. At about 12 o'clock, three muscles overlay this structure. From medial to lateral these are sternohyoid, omohyoid, and sternothyroid. Posterior to the thyroid cartilage is the epiglottis and the pharyngeal space. The superior aspect of the arytenoid cartilages can be seen posterior to the thyroid cartilage as well. Sternocleidomastoid sits at about 9 and 3 o'clock. All three scalenes and levator scapula can be seen from 9 to 7 o'clock. Postero-medially, trapezius begins to fan out. A corresponding CT scan captures the supraglottic structures quite well.

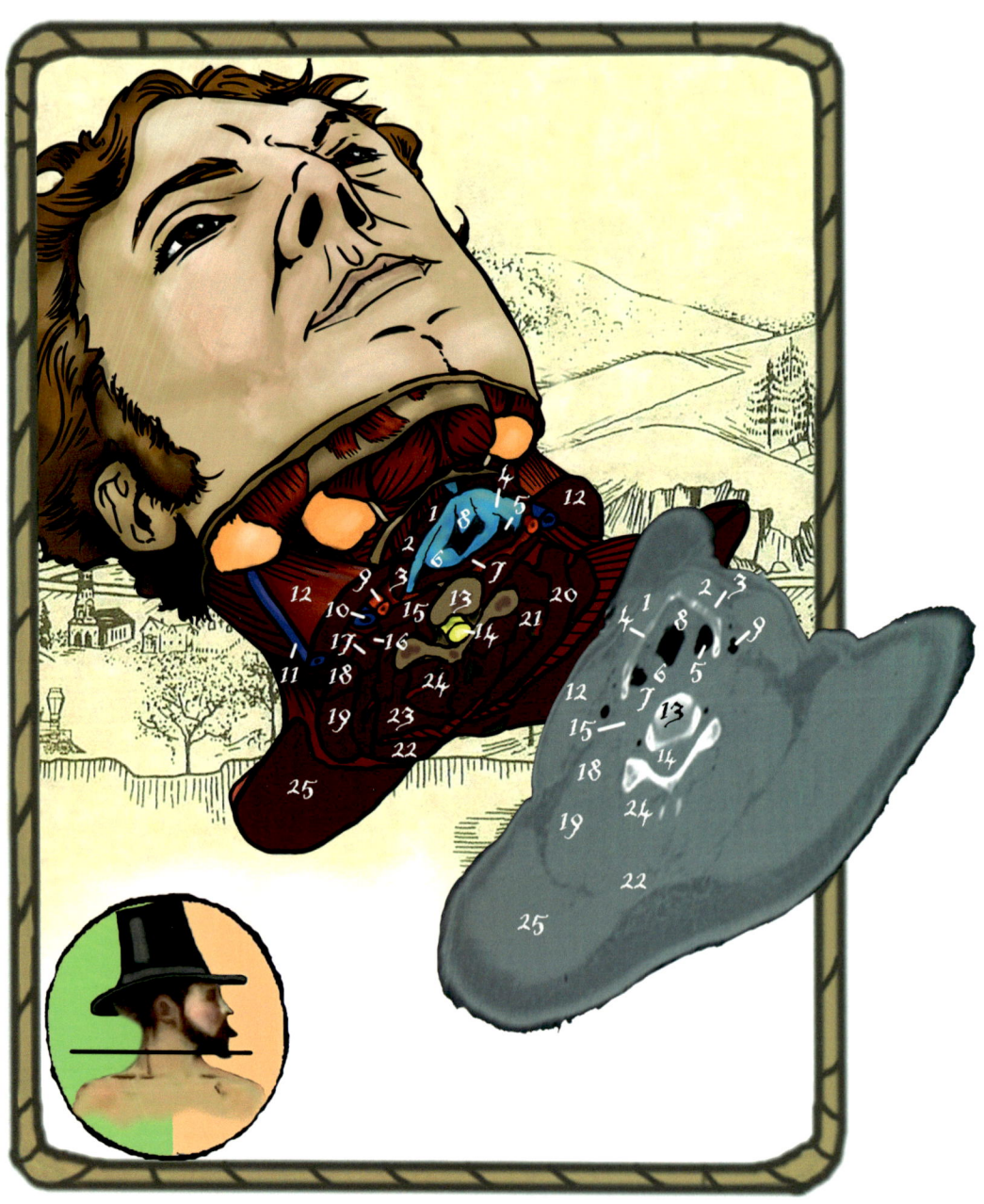

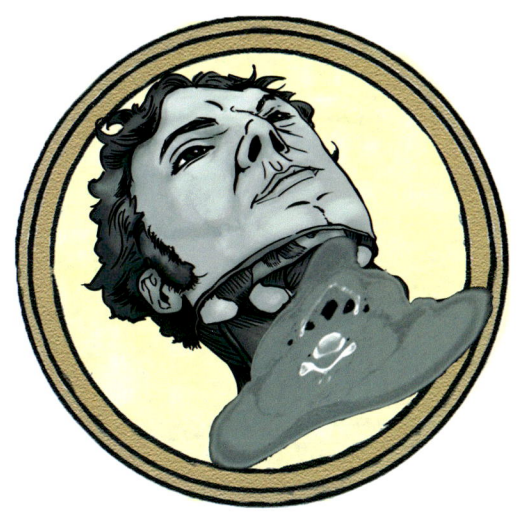

13. **Fifth cervical vertebra** (*Vertebra cervicale quinta*)

14. **Spinal Cord** (*Medulla spinalis*)

15. **Longus colli** (*M. longus colli*)

16. **Anterior scalene** (*M. scalenus anterior*) Derived from σκαληνός, meaning an irregular sided triangle, the muscles were named by Riolan in the 17th century.

17. **Middle scalene** (*M. scalenus medius*)

18. **Posterior scalene** (*M. scalenus posterior*)

19. **Levator scapulae** (*M. levator scapulae*)

20. **Longissimus cervicis** (*M. longissimus cervicis*)

21. **Longissimus capitis** (*M. longissimus capitis*)

22. **Splenius capitis** (*M. splenius capitis*) Derived from σπληνιου, meaning a bandage.

23. **Semispinalis capitis** (*M. semispinalis capitis*)

24. **Erector spinae** (*Musculus erector spinae*)

25. **Trapezius** (*M. trapezius*)

1. **Sternohyoid** (*M. sternohyoideus*)

2. **Omohyoid** (*M. omohyoideus*) Derived from ωμος, the term for shoulder, the muscle was named by Winslow in the 18th century.

3. **Sternothyroid** (*M. sternothyroideus*)

4. **Thyroid cartilage** (*Cartilago thyroidica*) Known colloquially as the Adam's apple, a term that first appeared during the 18th century.

5. **Pharynx** (*Pharynx*)

6. **Arytenoid cartilage** (*Cartilago arytenoidea*) Derived from ρυταινα, a term for a water pitcher, the cartilage was so named by Galen.

7. **Inferior pharyngeal constrictor** (*M. constrictor pharyngis inferior*)

8. **Epiglottis** (*Epiglottis*)

9. **Common carotid artery** (*Arteria carotis communis*)

10. **Internal jugular vein** (*Vena jugularis interna*)

11. **External jugular vein** (*Vena jugularis externa*)

12. **Sternocleidomastoid** (*M. sternocleidomastoideus*)

IX – The Rima Glottis – C – 6

The neck has been sliced at the inferior aspect of the thyroid cartilage to expose the cross-section of the rima glottis. The arytenoid cartilages are seen posterior to the rima glottis. Posterior to this structure is the inferior pharyngeal constrictor, which sits in close proximity to the body of the sixth cervical vertebra. The scalenes are here becoming more prominent, and trapezius is flaring out medially. The acromion process of the scapula may be appreciated on the left. A corresponding CT captures many of the structures radiographically.

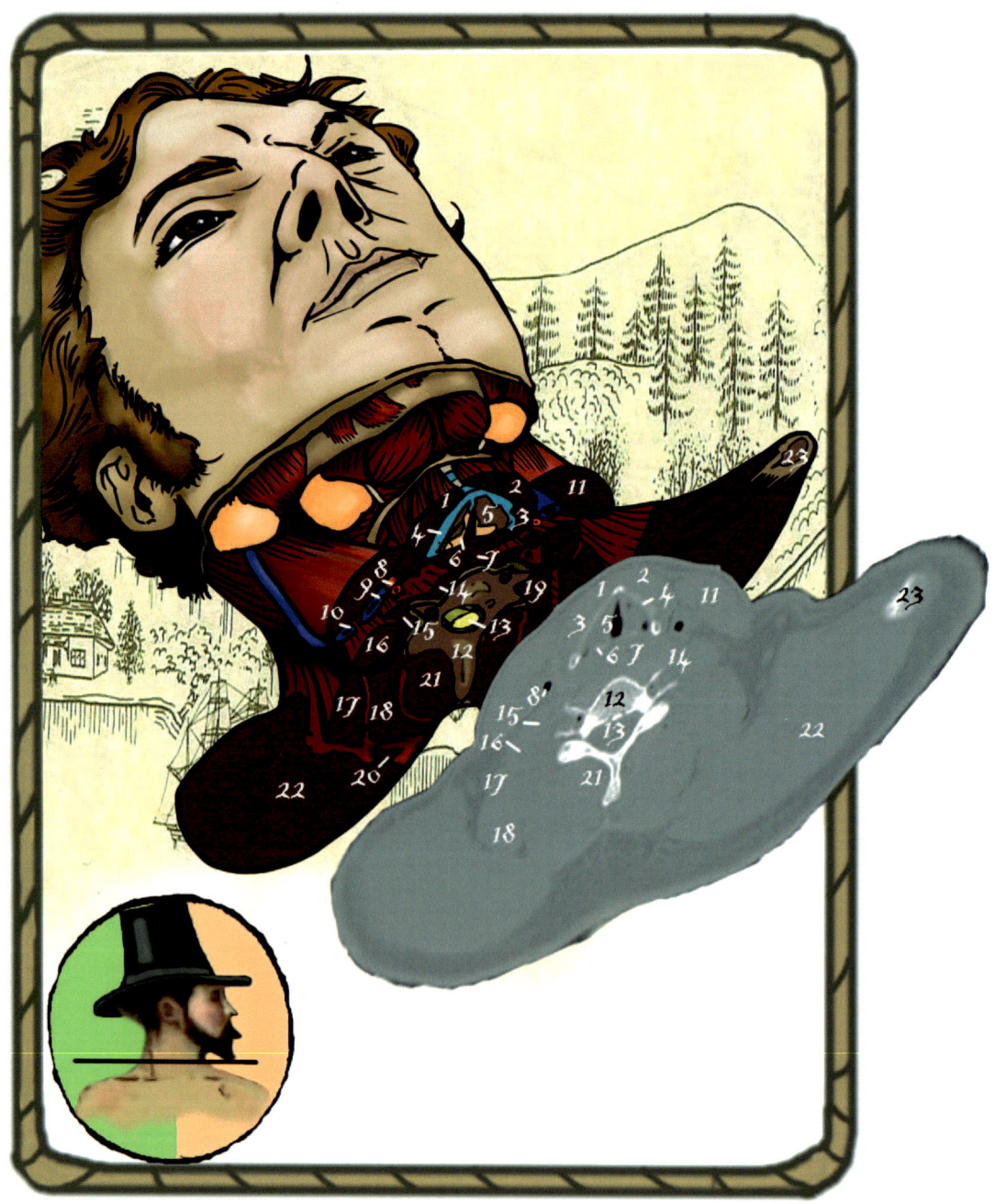

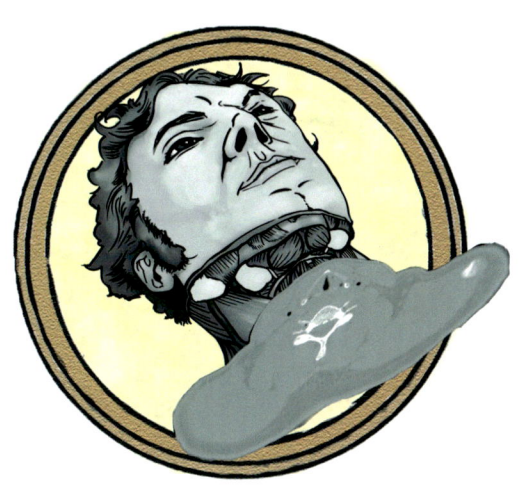

19. **Longissimus capitis** (*M. longissimus capitis*)

20. **Splenius capitis** (*M. splenius capitis*)

21. **Erector spinae** (*Musculus erector spinae*)

22. **Trapezius** (*M. trapezius*)

23. **Acromion process of the scapula** (*Scapula, acromion*) Derived from a combination of ακρου and ωμος, the terms for limb and shoulder, the bony process was named by Hippocrates.

1. **Sternohyoid** (*m. sternohyoideus*)

2. **Omohyoid** (*M. omohyoideus*)

3. **Sternothyroid** (*M. sternothyroideus*)

4. **Thyroid cartilage** (*Cartilago thyroidica*)

5. **Rima glottis** (*Rima glottidis*)

6. **Arytenoid cartilage** (*Cartilago arytenoidea*)

7. **Inferior pharyngeal constrictor** (*M. constrictor pharyngis inferior*)

8. **Common carotid artery** (*Arteria carotis communis*)

9. **Internal jugular vein** (*Vena jugularis interna*)

10. **External jugular vein** (*Vena jugularis externa*)

11. **Sternocleidomastoid** (*M. sternocleidomastoideus*)

12. **Sixth cervical vertebra** (*Vertebra cervicale sexta*)

13. **Spinal Cord** (*Medulla spinalis*)

14. **Longus colli** (*M. longus colli*)

15. **Anterior scalene** (*M. scalenus anterior*)

16. **Middle scalene** (*M. scalenus medius*)

17. **Posterior scalene** (*M. scalenus posterior*)

18. **Levator scapulae** (*M. levator scapulae*)

X – The Thyroid Gland – C-7

This section reveals the thyroid gland, a structure that sits in the midline straddling the cricoid cartilage. Note the overlying strap muscles, structures that must be carefully retracted while exposing the thyroid during surgery. Sternocleidomastoid has moved more medially, and is beginning to occlude the sternohyoid and sternothyroid strap muscles. Beneath the cricoid cartilage sits the oesophagus. The clavicle can be seen as well as the scapula and the surrounding scapular muscles. The corresponding CT scan captures these structures radiographically.

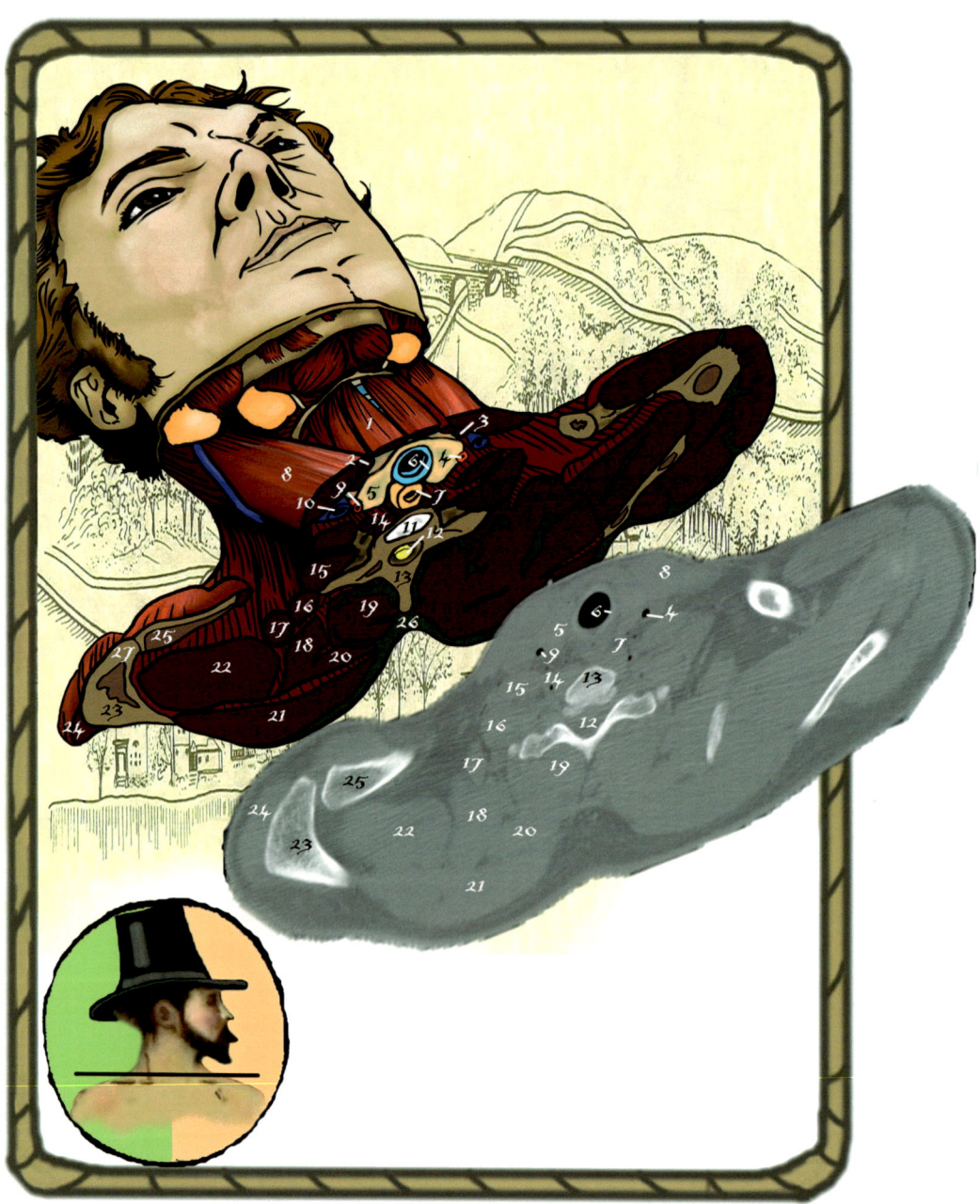

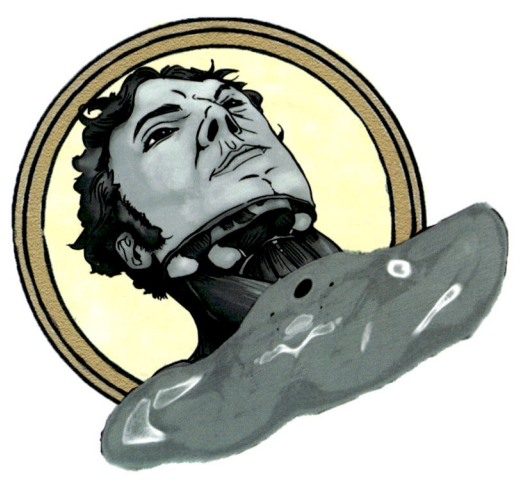

1. **Sternohyoid** (*M. sternohyoideus*)

2. **Omohyoid** (*M. omohyoideus*)

3. **Sternothyroid** (*M. sternothyroideus*)

4. **Left common carotid artery** (*Arteria carotis communis*)

5. **Thyroid gland** (*Glandulae thyroidea*) Derived from θυρεός, the large shields carried by Greek soldiers that covered the entire body to the neck, the gland was named by Galen.

6. **Cricoid cartilage** (*Cartilago cricoidea*) Derived from κρικος, meaning ring, the structure was named by the lexicographer Julius Pollux in the 2nd century.

7. **Oesophagus** (*Oesophagus*) Derived from οισοφάγος, the term for gullet.

8. **Sternocleidomastoid** (*M. sternocleidomastoideus*)

9. **Right common carotid artery** (*Arteria carotis communis*)

10. **Internal jugular vein** (*Vena jugularis interna*)

11. **Intervertebral disc** (*Discus intervertebralis*)

12. **Spinal Cord** (*Medulla spinalis*)

13. **Seventh cervical vertebra** (*Vertebra cervicale septima*)

14. **Longus colli** (*M. longus colli*)

15. **Anterior scalene** (*M. scalenus anterior*)

16. **Middle scalene** (*M. scalenus medius*)

17. **Posterior scalene** (*M. scalenus posterior*)

18. **Levator scapulae** (*M. levator scapulae*)

19. **Erector spinae** (*Musculus erector spinae*)

20. **Rhomboid minor** (*M. rhomboideus minor*)

21. **Trapezius** (*M. trapezius*)

22. **Supraspinatus** (*M. suprapinatus*)

23. **Scapula** (*Os scapula*)

24. **Deltoid** (*M. deltoideus*) Derived from Δ the fourth letter of the Greek alphabet, the muscle was named by Riolan in the 17th century.

25. **Clavicle** (*Clavicula*) Derived from κλείς, meaning key, the bone was described by Aristotle.

26. **Nuchal ligament** (*Lig. nuchae*) According to Skinner, the term is derived from nookah, the Arabic word for spine.

27. **Acromion process of the scapula** (*Scapula, acromion*)

XI – The Thoracic Inlet – T-2

In this section, the neck has been sliced at the level of the second thoracic vertebra, just superior to the level of the manubrium. The sternocleidomastoid muscles have coursed medially towards the midline, and their attachment on the clavicle is seen in cross section. Beneath the clavicle, at 12 o'clock, sits sternothyroid, and below these muscles can be seen the brachiocephalic veins as they turn into the subclavian veins. The left common carotid artery is seen medial to the left subclavian artery. The right brachiocephalic artery can be seen arching into the right subclavian artery. The trachea sits anterior to the oesophagus. Laterally, the deltoid muscle covers the superior aspect of the humerus. The glenohumeral joint may also seen. A CT corresponds nicely with many of these structures. Note the atelectasis and fluid collection in the posterior aspect of the lungs, the result of the CT being taken from a cadaver.

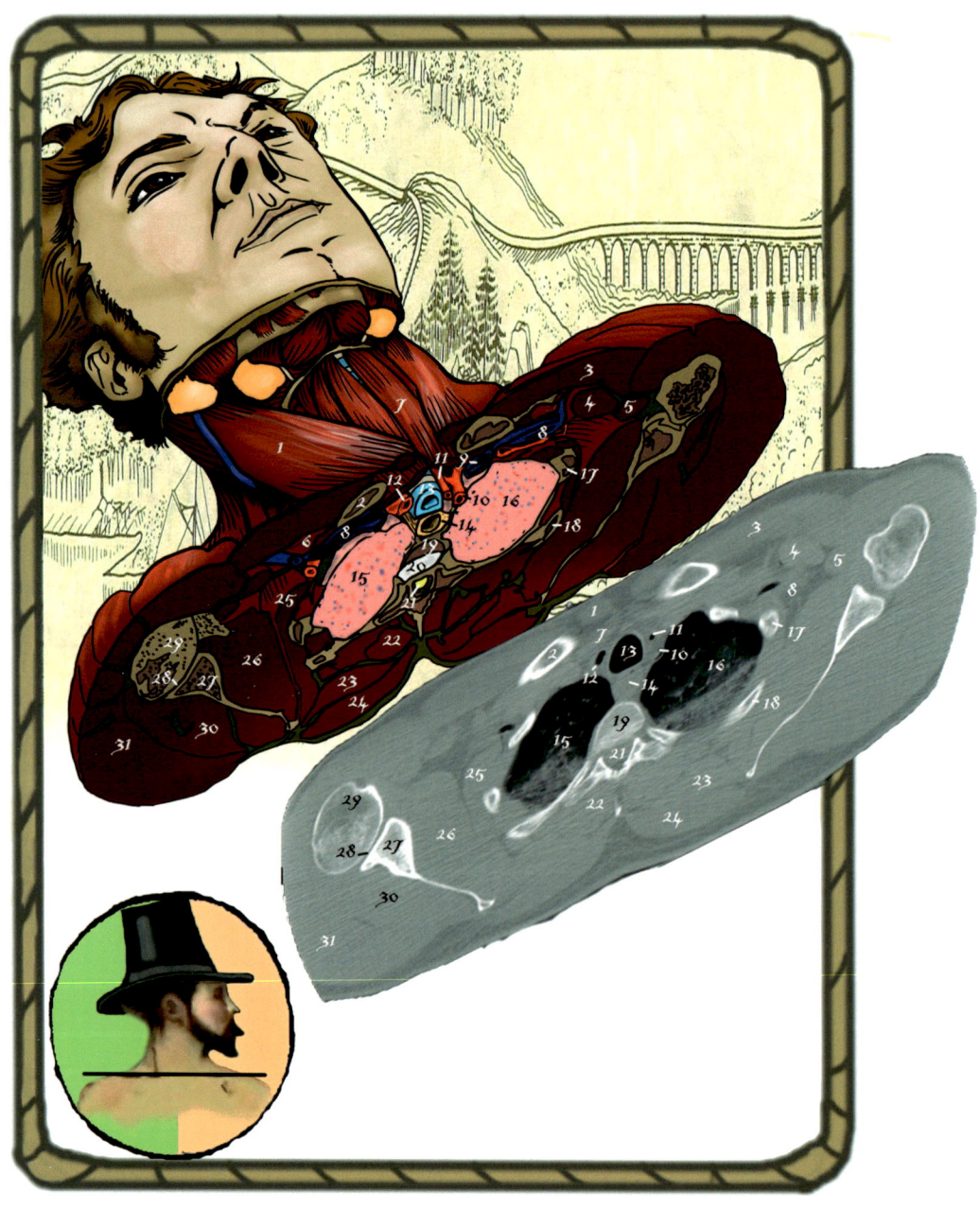

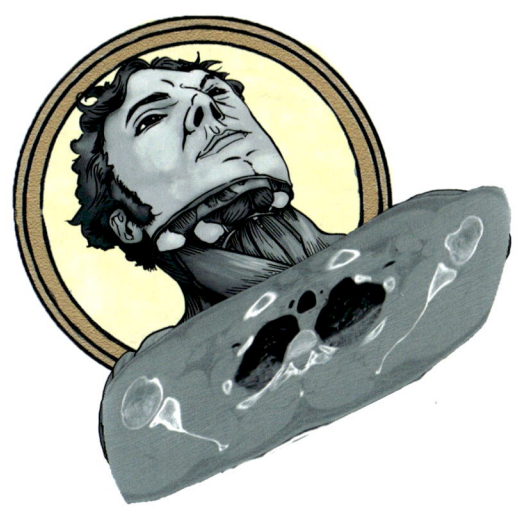

12. **Brachiocephalic artery** (*A. brachiocephalica*)

13. **Trachea** (*Trachea*)

14. **Oesophagus** (*Oesophagus*)

15. **Right lung** (*Pulmo dexter*)

16. **Left lung** (*Pulmo sinister*)

17. **First rib** (*Costa prima*)

18. **Second rib** (*Costa secunda*)

19. **Second thoracic vertebra** (*Vertebra thoracica secunda*)

20. **Intervertebral disc** (*Discus intervertebralis*)

21. **Spinal Cord** (*Medulla spinalis*)

22. **Erector spinae** (*Musculus erector spinae*)

23. **Rhomboid major** (*M. rhomboideus major*)

24. **Trapezius** (*M. trapezius*)

25. **Serratus anterior** (*M. serratus anterior*)

26. **Subscapularis** (*M. subscapularis*)

27. **Scapula** (*Os scapula*)

28. **Glenoid cavity** (*Cavitas glenoidalis*) Derived from γλήνη, meaning socket.

29. **Humerus** (*Humerus*)

30. **Infraspinatus** (*M. infraspinatus*)

31. **Deltoid** (*M. deltoideus*)

1. **Sternocleidomastoid** (*M. sternocleidomastoideus*)

2. **Clavicle** (*Clavicula*)

3. **Pectoralis major** (*M. pectoralis major*)

4. **Pectoralis minor** (*M. pectoralis minor*)

5. **Coracobrachialis** (*M. coracobrachialis*)

6. **Subscapularis** (*M. subscapularis*)

7. **Sternohyoid** (*M. sternothyroideus*)

8. **Subclavian vein** (*Vena subclavia*)

9. **Brachiocephalic vein** (*Vena brachiocephalica*)

10. **Subclavian artery** (*Arteria subclavia*)

11. **Left common carotid artery** (*Arteria carotis communis*)

CHAPTER TWO
THE THORAX

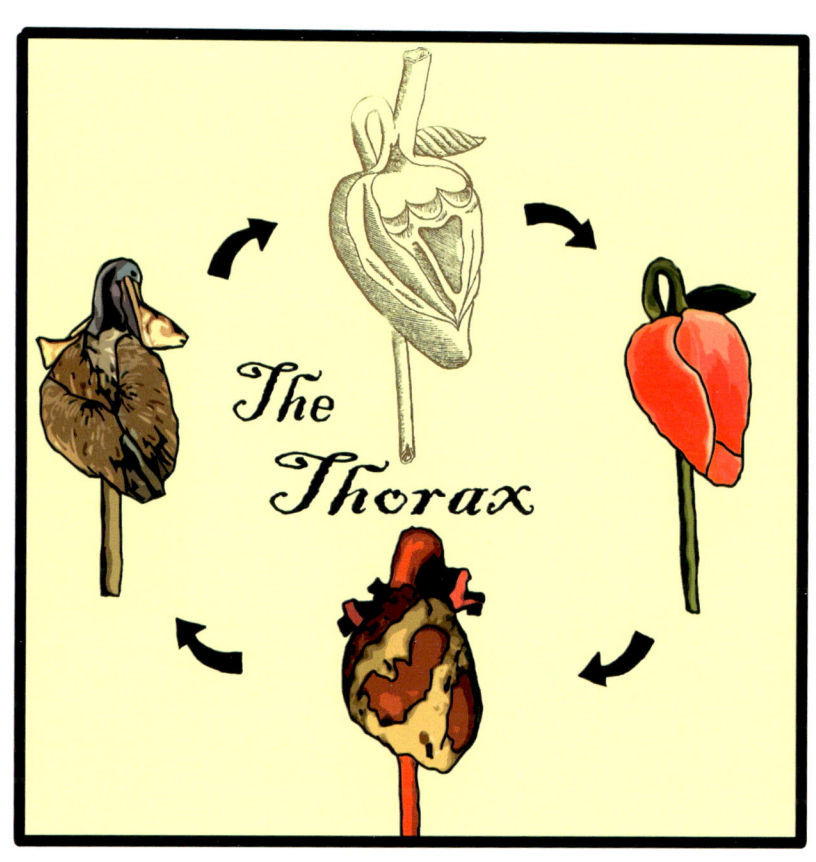

Part One:
The Male Thorax

I – Superior Thorax and Branches of the Great Vessels T – 3

The thorax, a term derived from θώραξ, a type of ancient Greek breast plate, was named by Hippocrates in the 5th century BC. In this section, the thorax has been sliced inferior to the clavicle and rotated to show mediastinal structures on the left. The three branches of the aorta, the brachiocephalic artery, the left common carotid artery, and the left subclavian artery, can be seen posterior to the left brachiocephalic vein, and anterior to the trachea and oesophagus. The left brachiocephalic vein is seen just superior to its merger with the right brachiocephalic vein to form the superior vena cava. A corresponding CT shows these structures radiographically.

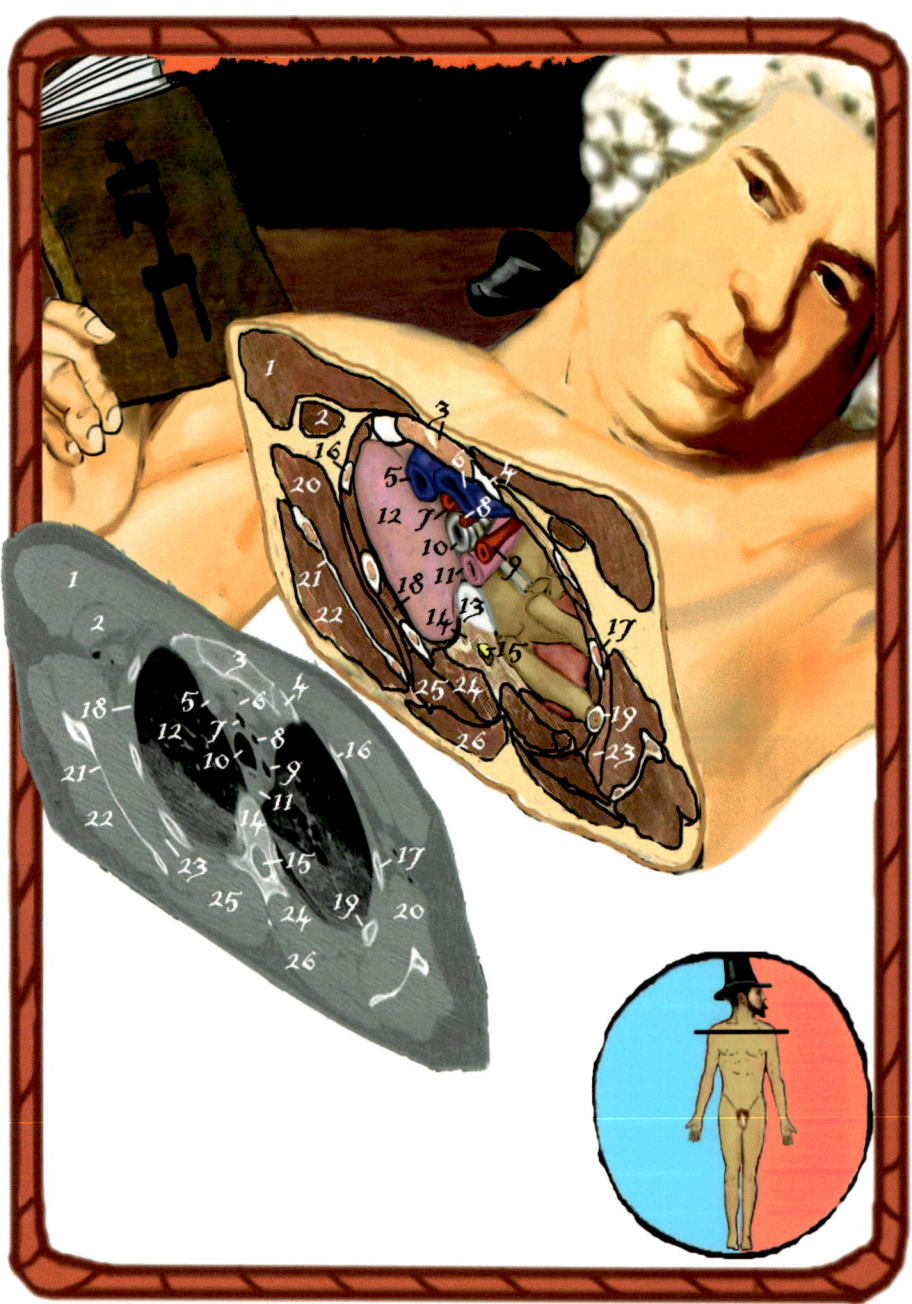

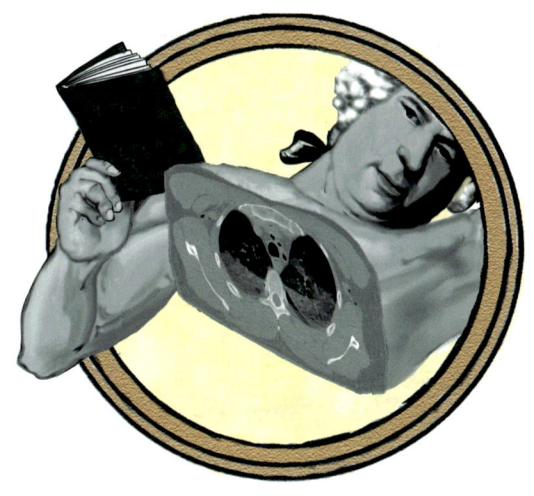

1. **Pectoralis major** (*M. pectoralis major*) Derived from pectoralis, a Roman breast plate, the muscles were named by Winslow, an 18th century Danish anatomist.

2. **Pectoralis minor** (*M. pectoralis minor*)

3. **Manubrium** (*Manubrium*) Derived from the Latin term for a handle, as in the handle of a sword, the bone was named by Vesalius.

4. **Costal cartilage of the first rib** (*Cartilago costalis*) The term costal is derived from the Latin term for rib, and was first used by Galen.

5. **Right brachiocephalic vein** (*Vena brachiocephalica*) The term vein is an anglicized form of the Latin vena, meaning vein. Skinner writes the term may come from the Latin verb venio, meaning to come, as blood comes to the heart through the veins.

6. **Left brachiocephalic vein** (*Vena brachiocephalica*)

7. **Brachiocephalic artery** (*Arteria brachiocephalica*) The term artery is derived from, αρτηρία, and means air duct. This term was used by the ancients as they believed arteries contained air. This is not an unreasonable conclusion, as when arteries were severed in carcasses, only air escaped, the blood having pooled in dependent veins.

8. **Left common carotid artery** (*Arteria carotis communis*)

9. **Left subclavian artery** (*Arteria subclavia*)

10. **Trachea** (*Trachea*) Derived from τραχεία, meaning rough, or the rough artery. The trachea was known to carry air, hence the term artery was used. It was originally described by Erasistratus in the 3rd century BC.

11. **Oesophagus** (*Oesophagus*)

12. **Superior lobe of the right lung** (*Pulmo dexter, lobus superior*) Derived from lunge, an Anglo-Saxon term meaning lightweight, their structure was first described by Malphigi in the 17th century.

13. **Intervertebral disc** (*Discus intervertebralis*) Derived from δίσκος, the term for a throwing discus, a popular sport in ancient Greece.

14. **Third thoracic vertebra** (*Vertebra thoracica tertia*)

15. **Spinal cord** (*Medulla spinalis*)

16. **First rib** (*Costa prima*)

17. **Second rib** (*Costa secunda*)

18. **Intercostal muscles** (*Mm. intercostales*)

19. **Third rib** (*Costa tertia*)

20. **Subscapularis** (*M. subscapularis*)

21. **Scapula** (*Scapula*) Derived from the Latin term for shoulder blade, the term was first used by Celsus in the 1st century.

22. **Infraspinatus** (*M. infraspinatus*)

23. **Serratus anterior** (*M. serratus anterior*)

24. **Erector spinae** (*M. erector spinae*)

25. **Rhomboid major** (*M. rhomboideus major*)

26. **Trapezius** (*M. trapezius*

II – Aortic Arch T- 4

In this section, the thorax has been sliced at T – 4, and rotated to show structures on the left. The aortic arch is prominently seen, occupying a position inferior to the thymus. The three main aortic branches, the brachiocephalic artery, the left common carotid artery, and the left subclavian artery, can be seen taking off at the superior aspect of the arch, with the trachea visible in the space between the brachiocephalic and left common carotid arteries. Further inferior, the trachea and oesophagus are medial to the aorta. A corresponding CT shows these structures radiographically.

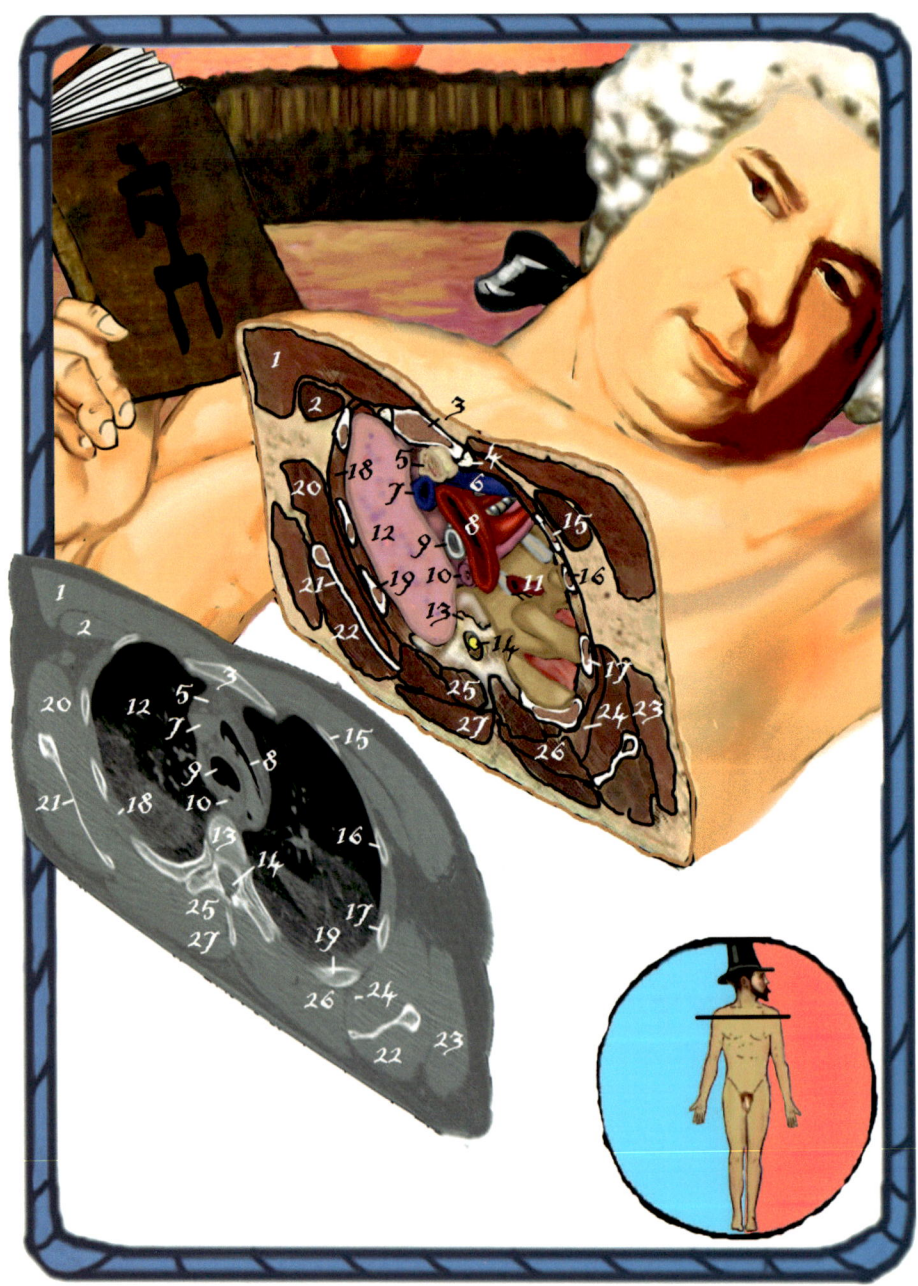

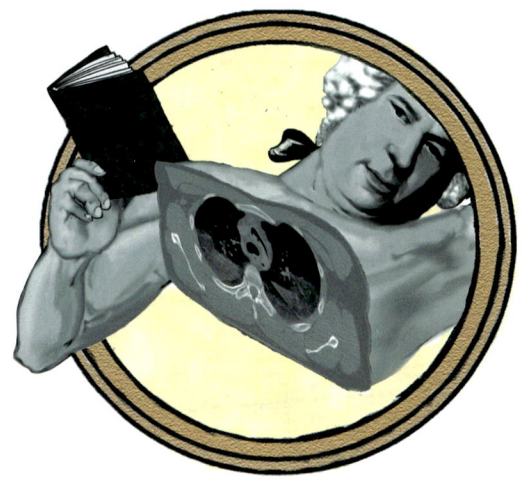

1. **Pectoralis major** (M. pectoralis major)

2. **Pectoralis minor** (M. pectoralis minor)

3. **Sternum** (Sternum) Derived from στέρνον, meaning specifically the male chest, the term was first used by Hippocrates.

4. **Costal cartilage of the first rib** (Cartilago costalis)

5. **Thymus** (Thymus) Derived from θύμος, the term for the herb thyme, the gland was first described by Berengarius in 16th century.

6. **Left brachiocephalic vein** (Vena brachio-cephalica)

7. **Superior vena cava** (Vena cava superior) Derived from the Latin term for hollow vein, the venae cavae were named by Diogenes due to the fact that they were often found empty in dissection specimens.

8. **Arch of aorta** (Arcus aortae) The term was first used by Aristotle, and it likely derives from the Greek term for the sheath of a sword, an object the ancient anatomists thought the vessel resembled.

9. **Trachea** (Trachea)

10. **Oesophagus** (Oesophagus)

11. **Left superior pulmonary vein** (Vena pulmo-nalis)

12. **Superior lobe of the right lung** (Pulmo dexter, lobus superior)

13. **Fourth thoracic vertebra** (Vertebra thoracica quarta)

14. **Spinal cord** (Medulla spinalis)

15. **Second rib** (Costa secunda)

16. **Third rib** (Costa tertia)

17. **Fourth rib** (Costa quarta)

18. **Intercostal muscles** (Mm. intercostales)

19. **Fifth rib** (Costa quinta)

20. **Subscapularis** (M. subscapularis)

21. **Scapula** (Scapula)

22. **Infraspinatus** (M. infraspinatus)

23. **Latissimus dorsi** (M. Latissimus dorsi)

24. **Serratus anterior** (M. serratus anterior)

25. **Erector spinae** (M. erector spinae)

26. **Rhomboid minor** (M. rhomboideus minor)

27. **Trapezius** (M. trapezius)

III – Azygos Arch T – 5

In this section, the thorax has been sliced at T-5 and rotated to show structures on the left. The thymus sits at 12 o'clock anterior to the superior vena cava and the ascending aorta. The aortic arch is slightly left of the midline, with descending aorta sitting just to the left of the fifth thoracic vertebra. The left brachiocephalic vein sits posterior to the three main aortic branches. The trachea sits anterior to the oesophagus in the midline. A corresponding CT shows these structures radiographically.

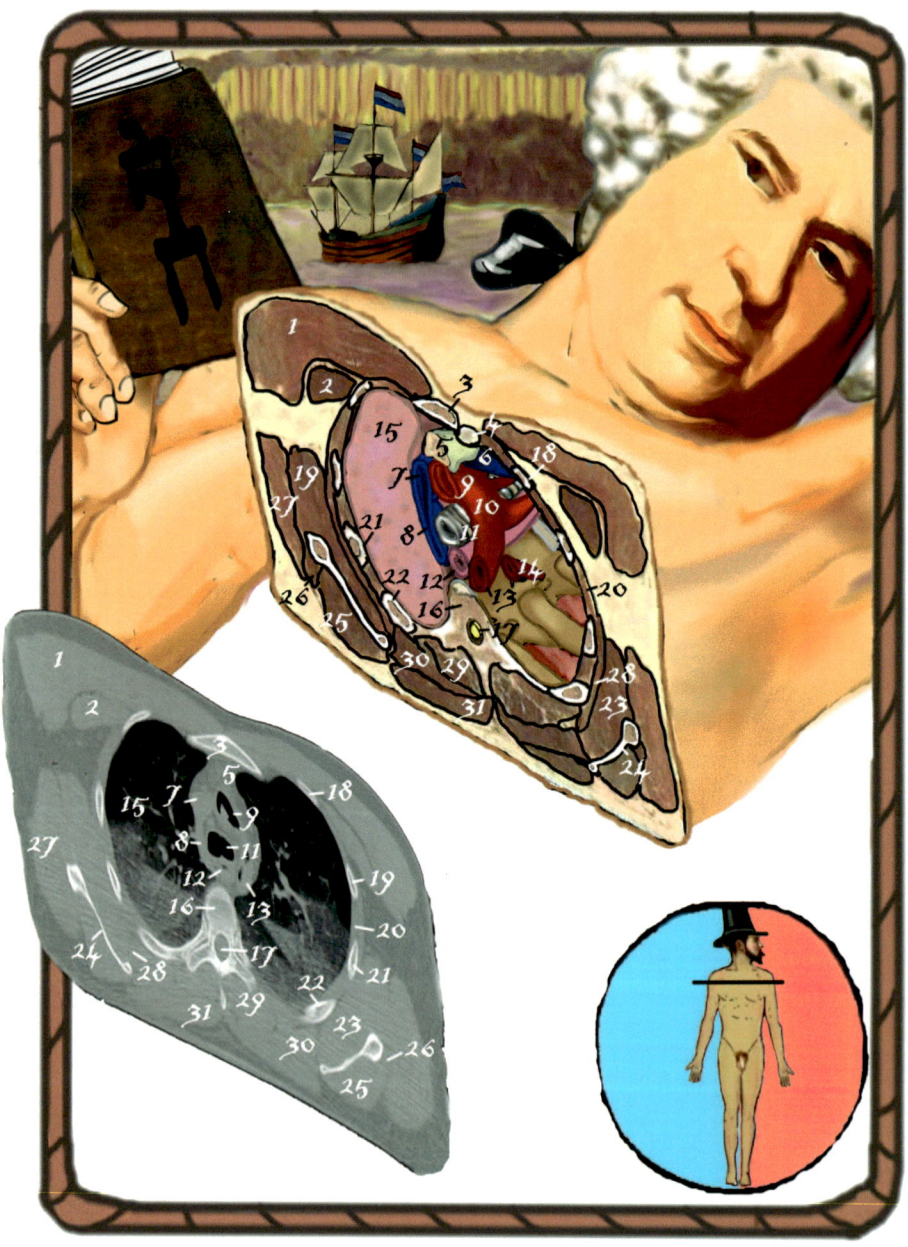

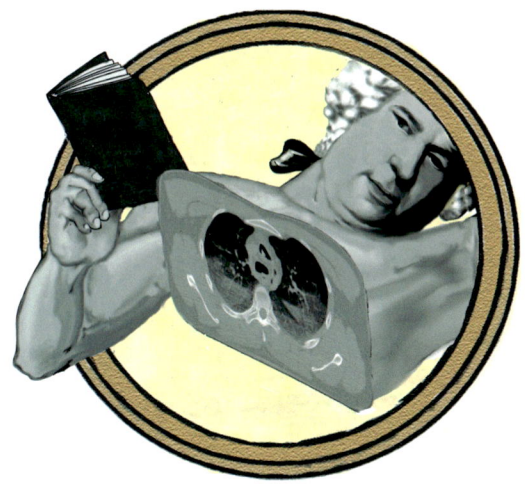

18. **Second rib** (Costa secunda)

19. **Third rib** (Costa tertia)

20. **Intercostal muscles** (Mm. intercostales)

21. **Fourth rib** (Costa quarta)

22. **Fifth rib** (Costa quinta)

23. **Subscapularis** (M. subscapularis)

24. **Scapula** (Scapula)

25. **Infraspinatus** (M. infraspinatus)

26. **Teres minor** (M. teres minor) Derived from the Latin term for round, the muscles were named by Cowper in the 18th century.

27. **Latissimus dorsi** (M. Latissimus dorsi)

28. **Serratus anterior** (M. serratus anterior)

29. **Erector spinae** (M. erector spinae)

30. **Rhomboid minor** (M. rhomboideus minor)

31. **Trapezius** (M. trapezius)

1. **Pectoralis major** (M. pectoralis major)

2. **Pectoralis minor** (M. pectoralis minor)

3. **Sternum** (Sternum).

4. **Costal cartilage of the first rib** (Cartilago costalis)

5. **Thymus** (Thymus)

6. **Left brachiocephalic vein** (Vena brachiocephalica)

7. **Superior vena cava** (Vena cava superior)

8. **Arch of the azygos vein** (Arcus venae azygos) Derived from, αζυξ, meaning unpaired, the vein was named by Galen in the 2nd century.

9. **Ascending aorta** (Aorta ascendens)

10. **Arch of aorta** (Arcus aortae)

11. **Trachea** (Trachea)

12. **Oesophagus** (Oesophagus)

13. **Descending aorta** (Aorta descendens)

14. **Left superior pulmonary vein** (Vena pulmonalis)

15. **Superior lobe of the right lung** (Pulmo dexter, lobus superior)

16. **Fifth thoracic vertebra** (Vertebra thoracica quinta)

17. **Spinal cord** (Medulla spinalis)

III – Azygos Arch T – 5

In this section, the thorax has been sliced at T-5, and rotated to show structures on the right. The thymus sits in the midline, posterior to the sternum and anterior to the aortic arch and superior vena cava. The arch of the azygos vein is seen as it extends posteriorly from the spinal column to merge with the posterior aspect of the superior vena cava. The trachea and oesophagus occupy the midline, while the arched aorta is seen on the left. A corresponding CT shows these structures radiographically.

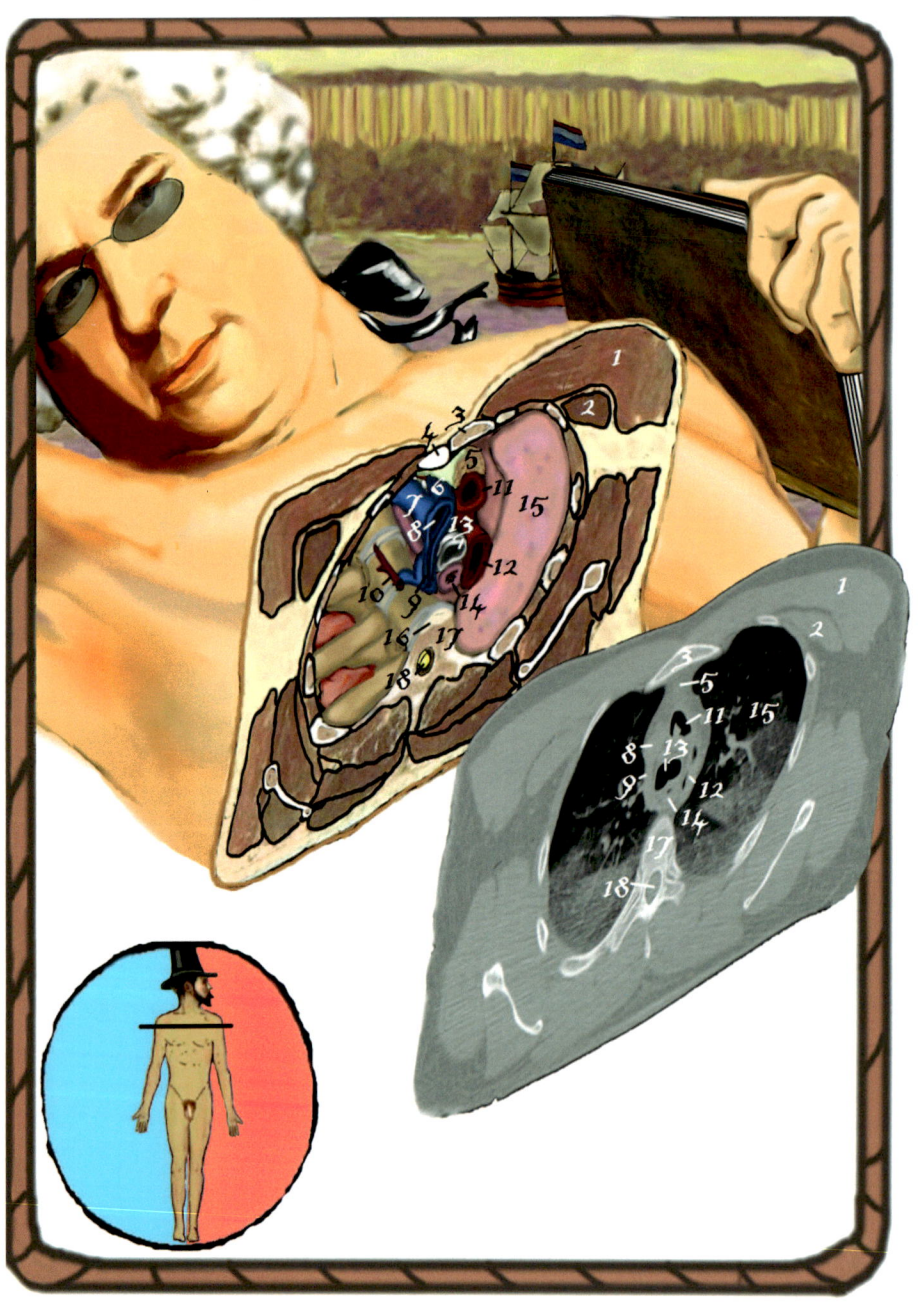

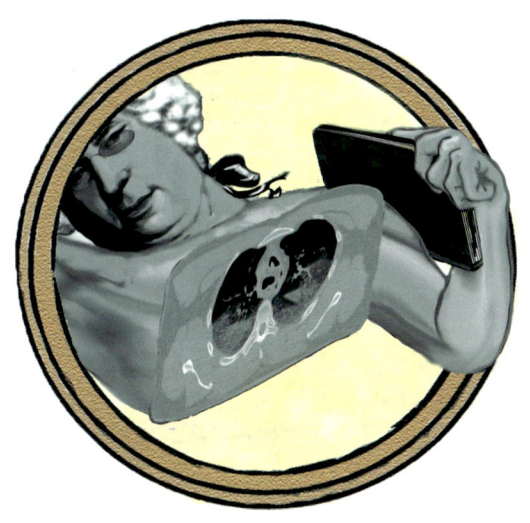

13. **Trachea** (Trachea)

14. **Oesophagus** (Oesophagus)

15. **Superior lobe of the right lung** (Pulmo dexter, lobus superior)

16. **Intervertebral disc** (Discus intervertebralis)

17. **Fifth thoracic vertebra** (Vertebra thoracica quinta)

18. **Spinal cord** (Medulla spinalis)

1. **Pectoralis major** (M. pectoralis major)

2. **Pectoralis minor** (M. pectoralis minor)

3. **Sternum** (Sternum)

4. **Costal cartilage of the first rib** (Cartilago costalis)

5. **Thymus** (Thymus)

6. **Left brachiocephalic vein** (Vena brachiocephalica)

7. **Right brachiocephalic vein** (Vena brachiocephalica)

8. **Superior vena cava** (Vena cava superior)

9. **Arch of the azygos vein** (Arcus venae azygos)

10. **Right superior pulmonary vein** (Vena pulmonalis)

11. **Ascending aorta** (Aorta ascendens)

12. **Descending aorta** (Aorta descendens)

IV – Superior Pulmonary Artery T – 5

In this section, the thorax has been sliced at T-5, and rotated to show structures on the left. The thymus sits in the midline slightly posterior to the sternum. Note the relation of the aortic arch to the superiormost aspect of the left pulmonary artery, as this latter structure fits snugly in the concavity of the former. Anterior to the distal end of the left pulmonary artery sits a branch of the left superior pulmonary vein. The left and right main bronchi straddle the midline anterior to the oesophagus and the azygos vein. A corresponding CT shows these structures radiographically.

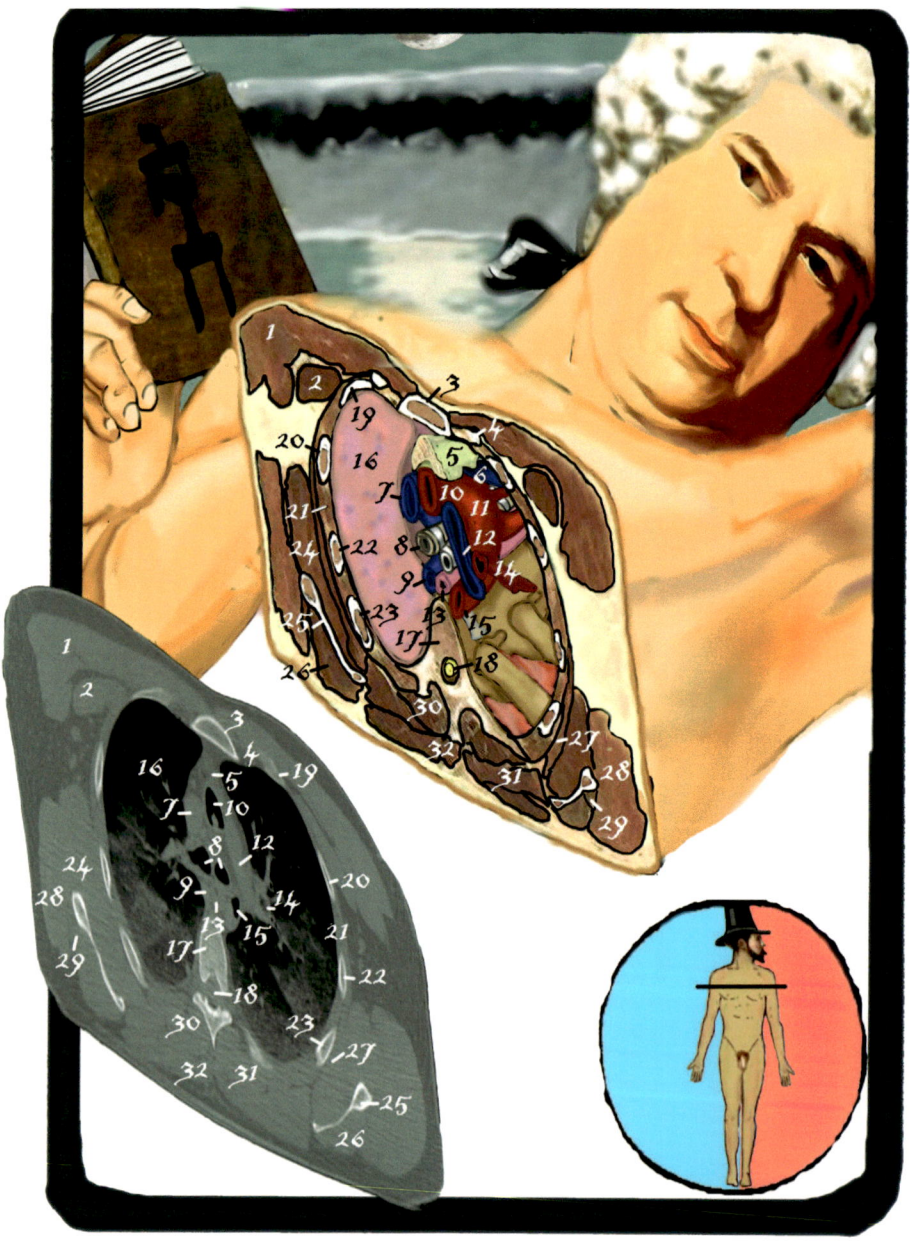

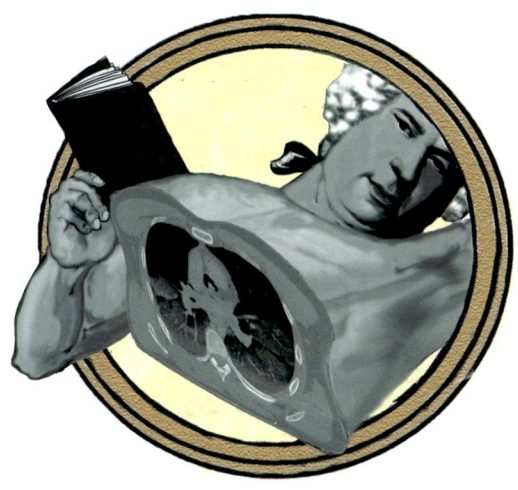

17. **Fifth thoracic vertebra** (Vertebra thoracica quinta)

18. **Spinal cord** (Medulla spinalis)

19. **Second rib** (Costa secunda)

20. **Third rib** (Costa tertia)

21. **Intercostal muscles** (Mm. intercostales)

22. **Fourth rib** (Costa quarta)

23. **Fifth rib** (Costa quinta)

24. **Subscapularis** (M. subscapularis)

25. **Scapula** (Scapula)

26. **Infraspinatus** (M. infraspinatus)

27. **Serratus anterior** (M. serratus anterior)

28. **Teres major** (M. teres major)

29. **Latissimus dorsi** (M. Latissimus dorsi)

30. **Erector spinae** (M.erector spinae)

31. **Rhomboid major** (M. rhomboideus major)

32. **Trapezius** (M. trapezius)

1. **Pectoralis major** (M. pectoralis major)

2. **Pectoralis minor** (M. pectoralis minor)

3. **Sternum** (Sternum)

4. **Costal cartilage of the second rib** (Cartilago costalis)

5. **Thymus** (Thymus)

6. **Left brachiocephalic vein** (Vena brachio-cephalica)

7. **Superior vena cava** (Vena cava superior)

8. **Right and left main bronchi** (Bronchus) Derived from βρόγχοσ, the term originates from the verb to moisten, as the ancients believed the bronchi were the structures that delivered liquids to the stomach. The oesophagus was for solids.

9. **Azygos vein** (Vena azygos)

10. **Ascending aorta** (Aorta ascendens)

11. **Arch of aorta** (Arcus aortae)

12. **Left pulmonary artery** (Arteria pulmonalis)

13. **Oesophagus** (Oesophagus)

14. **Left superior pulmonary vein** (Vena pulmonalis)

15. **Descending aorta** (Aorta descendens)

16. **Superior lobe of the right lung** (Pulmo dexter, lobus superior)

V – The Pulmonary Trunk T – 5

In this section, the thorax has been sliced at T -5 and rotated to show structures on the left. The thymus sits at 12 o'clock posterior to the sternum. The ascending aorta sits posterior to this structure with the pulmonary trunk occupying the space in its concavity. The pulmonary trunk bifurcates into the left and right pulmonary arteries, vessels that are anterior to the right and left main bronchi. The descending aorta, oesophagus, and the azygos vein are more posterior. A corresponding CT shows these structures radiographically.

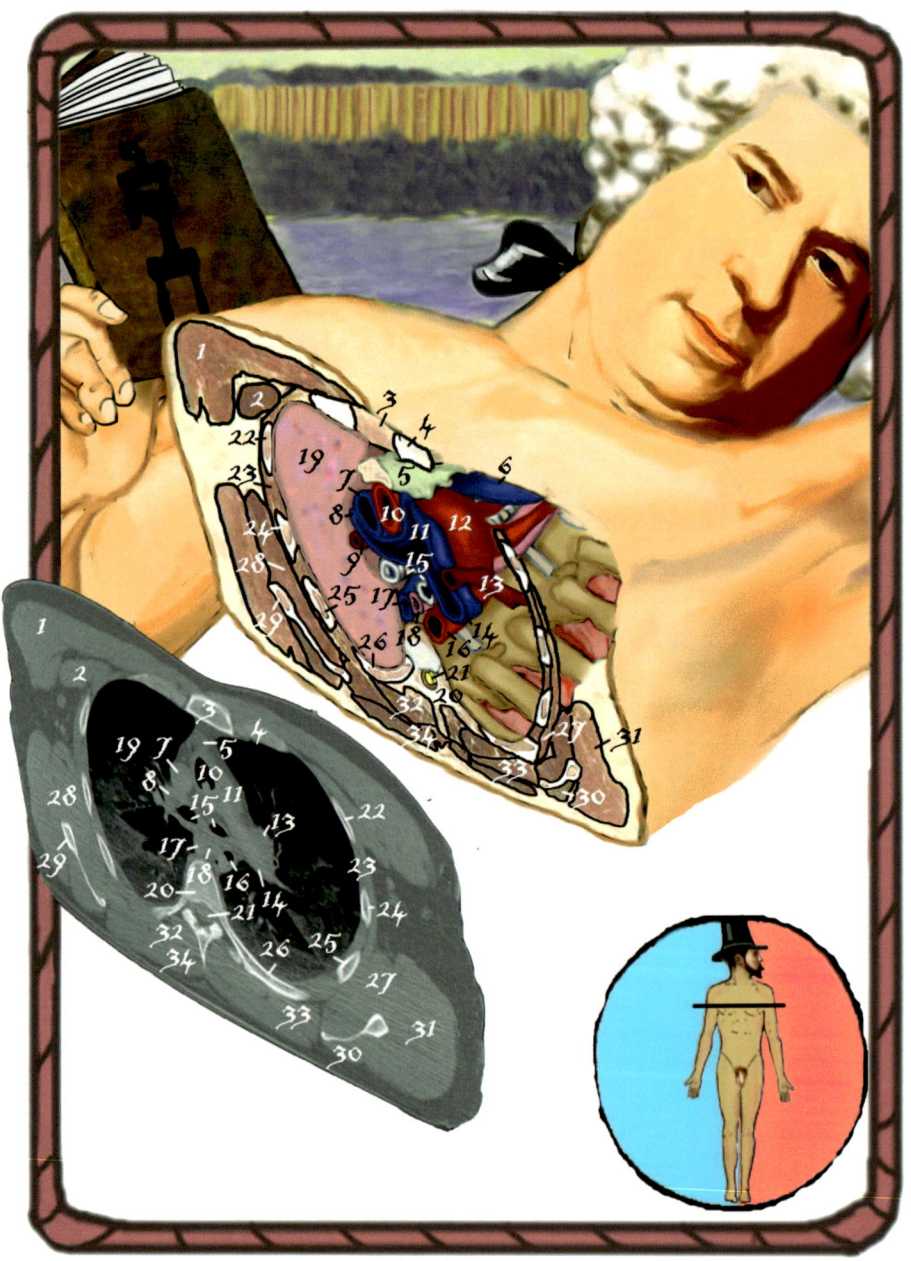

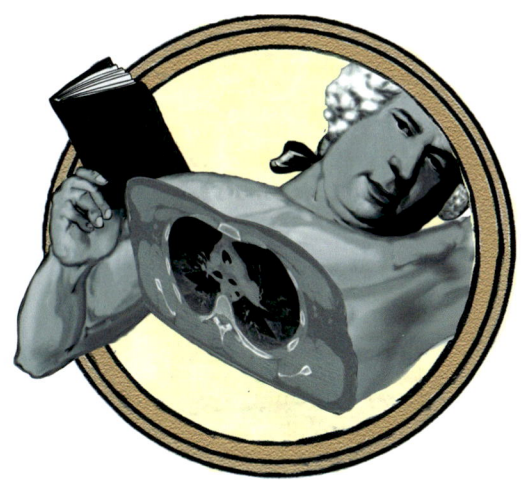

1. **Pectoralis major** (M. pectoralis major)

2. **Pectoralis minor** (M. pectoralis minor)

3. **Sternum** (Sternum)

4. **Costal cartilage of the second rib** (Cartilago costalis)

5. **Thymus** (Thymus)

6. **Left brachiocephalic vein** (Vena brachiocephalica)

7. **Superior vena cava** (Vena cava superior)

8. **Right pulmonary artery** (Arteria pulmonalis)

9. **Right superior pulmonary vein** (Vena pulmonalis)

10. **Ascending aorta** (Aorta ascendens)

11. **Pulmonary trunk** (Truncus pulmonalis) Derived from pulmo, the Latin term for lung, the term was first applied to the pulmonary arteries and veins by Malphigi in the 17th century.

12. **Arch of aorta** (Arcus aortae)

13. **Left superior pulmonary vein** (Vena pulmonalis)

14. **Left pulmonary artery** (Arteria pulmonalis)

15. **Left and right main bronchi** (Bronchus)

16. **Descending aorta** (Aorta descendens)

17. **Azygos vein** (Vena azygos)

18. **Oesophagus** (Oesophagus)

19. **Superior lobe of the right lung** (Pulmo dexter, lobus superior) Derived from lunge, an Anglo-Saxon term meaning lightweight, their structure was first described by Malphigi in the 17th century.

20. **Fifth thoracic vertebra** (Vertebra thoracica quinta)

21. **Spinal cord** (Medulla spinalis)

22. **Third rib** (Costa tertia)

23. **Intercostal muscles** (Mm. intercostales)

24. **Fourth rib** (Costa quarta)

25. **Fifth rib** (Costa quinta)

26. **Sixth rib** (Costa sexta)

27. **Serratus anterior** (M. serratus anterior)

28. **Subscapularis** (M. subscapularis)

29. **Scapula** (Scapula)

30. **Infraspinatus** (M. infraspinatus)

31. **Latissimus dorsi** (M. Latissimus dorsi)

32. **Erector spinae** (M. erector spinae)

33. **Rhomboid major** (M. rhomboideus major)

34. **Trapezius** (M. trapezius)

V – The Pulmonary Trunk T – 5

In this section, the thorax has been sliced at T -5 and rotated to show structures on the right. The thymus sits just posterior to the sternum. Posterior to the thymus, the lumens of the superior vena cava, the ascending aorta, and the pulmonary trunk sit on an almost parallel line that runs from about 10 to 2 o'clock. The pulmonary trunk bifurcates into the left and right pulmonary arteries, the latter artery occupying a space between the right main bronchus and the superior vena cava. Note how the azygos vein arches over the right main bronchus. The oesophagus occupies a place in the midline. A corresponding CT shows these structures radiographically.

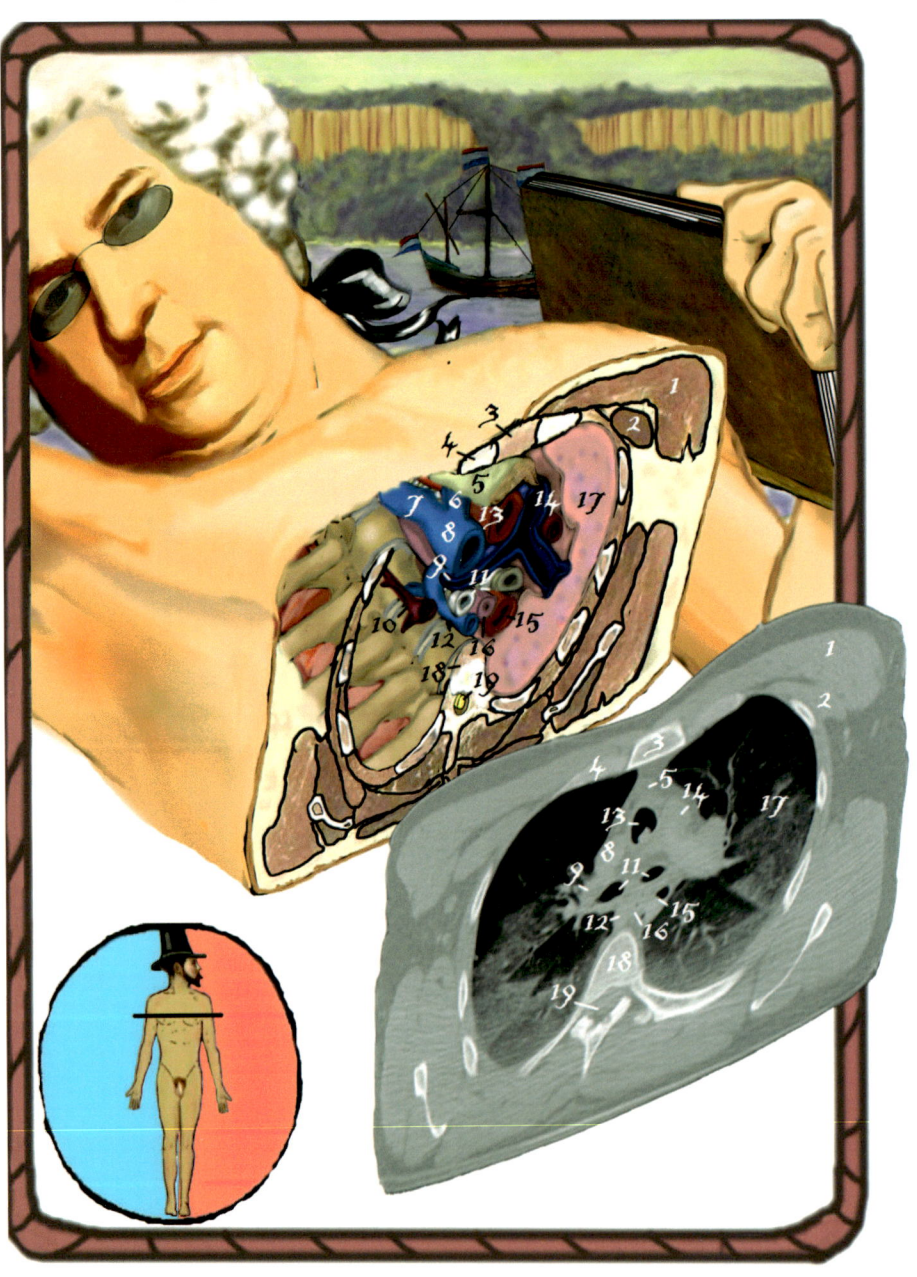

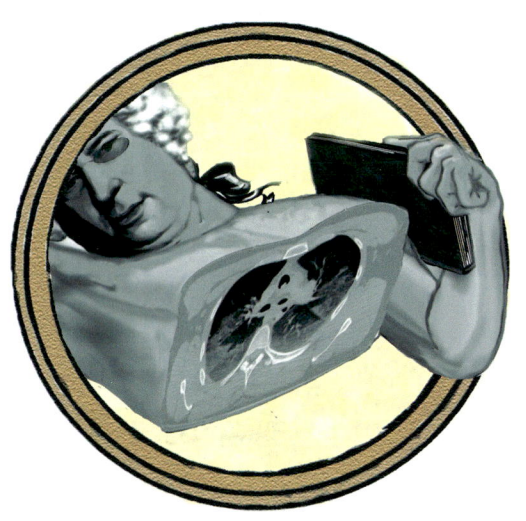

18. **Fifth thoracic vertebra** (Vertebra thoracica quinta)

19. **Spinal cord** (Medulla spinalis)

1. **Pectoralis major** (M. pectoralis major)

2. **Pectoralis minor** (M. pectoralis minor)

3. **Sternum** (Sternum)

4. **Costal cartilage of the second rib** (Cartilago costalis)

5. **Thymus** (Thymus)

6. **Left brachiocephalic vein** (Vena brachio-cephalica)

7. **Right brachiocephalic vein** (Vena brachio-cephalica)

8. **Superior vena cava** (Vena cava superior)

9. **Right pulmonary artery** (Arteria pulmona-lis)

10. **Right superior pulmonary vein** (Vena pul-monalis)

11. **Right and left main bronchi** (Bronchus)

12. **Azygos vein** (Vena azygos)

13. **Ascending aorta** (Aorta ascendens)

14. **Pulmonary trunk** (Truncus pulmonalis)

15. **Descending aorta** (Aorta descendens)

16. **Oesophagus** (Oesophagus)

17. **Superior lobe of the left lung** (Pulmo dexter, lobus superior)

VI – The Left Atrium T – 6

In this section, the thorax has been sliced at T-6 and rotated to show structures on the left. The thymus sits beneath the sternum. The lumen of the pulmonary trunk can be traced from its opening in the right ventricle to its bifurcation into the left and right pulmonary arteries. The lumen of the aorta is seen posterior to the pulmonary trunk, and this can be traced to the aortic arch and descending aorta. The left pulmonary veins empty into the left ventricle. A corresponding CT shows these structures radiographically.

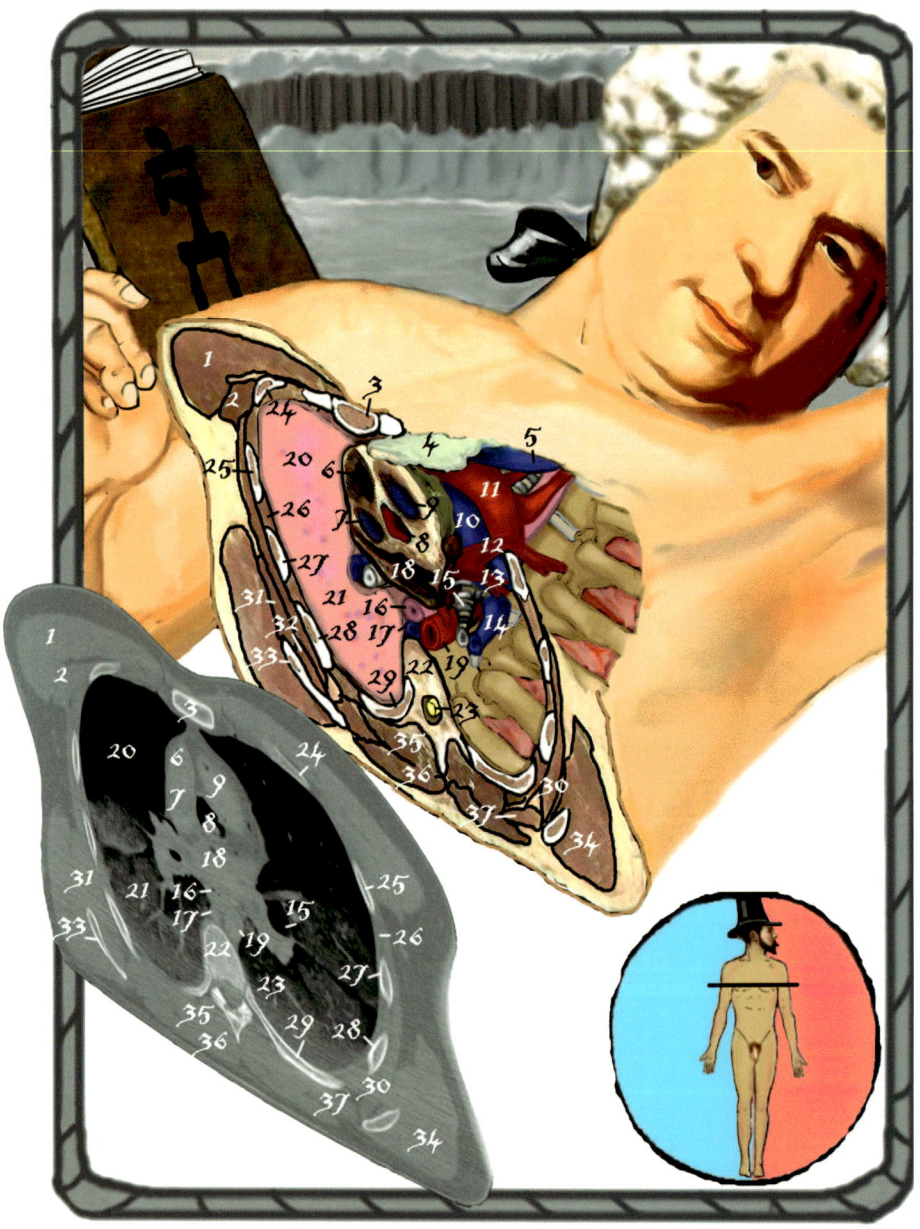

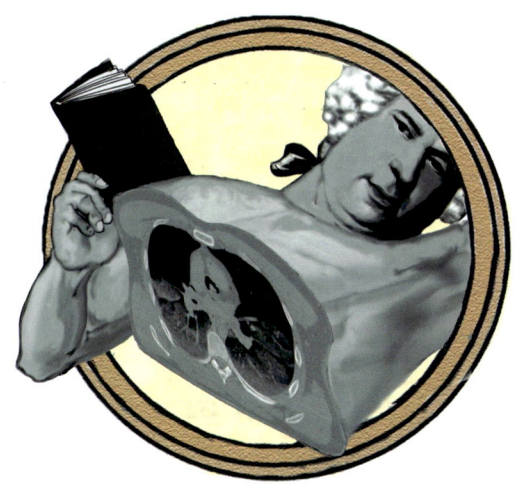

1. **Pectoralis major** (M. pectoralis major)
2. **Pectoralis minor** (M. pectoralis minor)
3. **Sternum** (Sternum)
4. **Thymus** (Thymus)
5. **Left brachiocephalic vein** (Vena brachio-cephalica)
6. **Right atrium** (Atrium dextrum) The term atrium is derived from the Latin word for courtyard, or the centrally located open part of a Roman house.
7. **Superior vena cava** (Vena cava superior)
8. **Ascending aorta** (Aorta ascendens)
9. **Right ventricle** (Ventriculus dexter)
10. **Pulmonary trunk** (Truncus pulmonalis)
11. **Arch of aorta** (Arcus aortae)
12. **Left superior pulmonary vein** (Vena pulmonalis)
13. **Left middle pulmonary vein** (Vena pulmonalis)
14. **Left pulmonary artery** (Arteria pulmonalis)
15. **Left inferior lobar bronchus** (Bronchus lobaris inferior sinister)
16. **Oesophagus** (Oesophagus)
17. **Azygos vein** (Vena azygos)

18. **Left atrium** (Atrium sinistrum)
19. **Descending aorta** (Aorta descendens)
20. **Superior lobe of the right lung** (Pulmo dexter, lobus superior)
21. **Middle lobe of the right lung** (Pulmo dexter, lobus medius)
22. **Sixth thoracic vertebra** (Vertebra thoracica sexta)
23. **Spinal cord** (Medulla spinalis)
24. **Third rib** (Costa tertia)
25. **Fourth rib** (Costa quarta)
26. **Intercostal muscles** (Mm. intercostales)
27. **Fifth rib** (Costa quinta)
28. **Sixth rib** (Costa sexta)
29. **Seventh rib** (Costa septima)
30. **Serratus anterior** (M. serratus anterior)
31. **Teres major** (M. teres major)
32. **Subscapularis** (M. subscapularis)
33. **Scapula** (Scapula)
34. **Latissimus dorsi** (M. Latissimus dorsi)
35. **Erector spinae** (M. erector spinae)
36. **Trapezius** (M. trapezius)
37. **Rhomboid major** (M. rhomboideus major)

VI – The Superior Vena Cava and the Right Atrium T – 6

In this section, the thorax has been sliced at T-6 and rotated to show structures on the right. The thymus sits askew of the midline, between 11 and 12 o'clock, posterior to the sternum. The left and right brachiocephalic veins are seen merging into the superior vena cava. The lumen of this latter structure is seen in cross-section just before it empties into the right atrium. Posterior to the superior vena cava is a branch of the right pulmonary artery and the superior right bronchus. The right superior pulmonary vein is seen as it empties into the left atrium. A corresponding CT shows these structures radiographically.

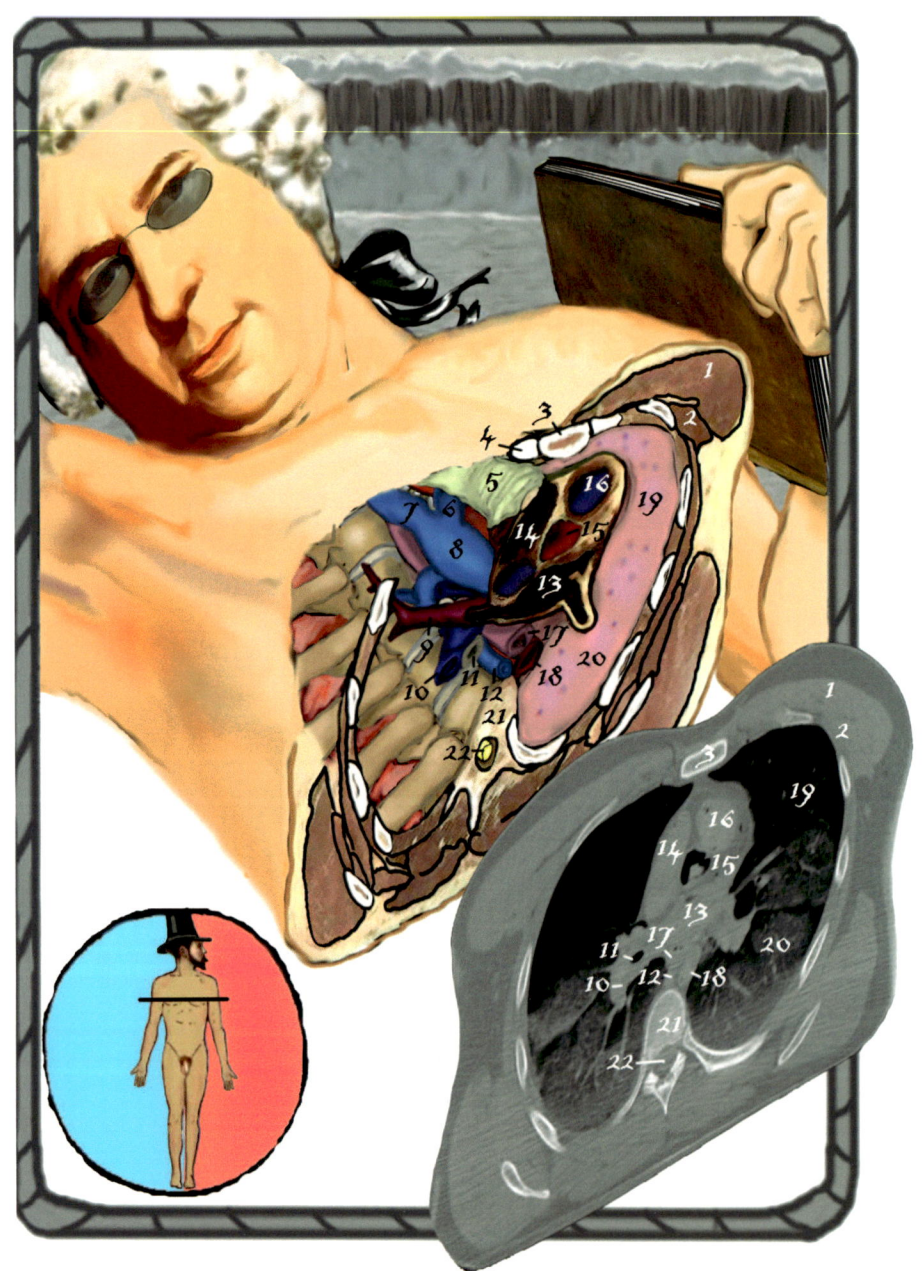

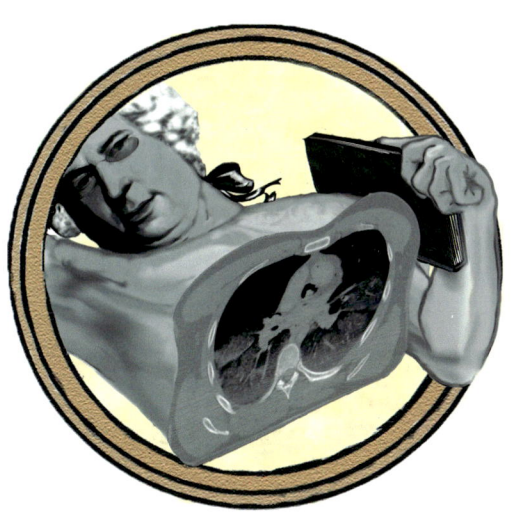

19. **Superior lobe of the left lung** (Pulmo sinister, lobus superior)

20. **Inferior lobe of the left lung** (Pulmo sinister, lobus inferior)

21. **Sixth thoracic vertebra** (Vertebra thoracica sexta)

22. **Spinal cord** (Medulla spinalis)

1. **Pectoralis major** (M. pectoralis major)

2. **Pectoralis minor** (M. pectoralis minor)

3. **Sternum** (Sternum)

4. **Costal cartilage of the third rib** (Cartilago costalis)

5. **Thymus** (Thymus)

6. **Left brachiocephalic vein** (Vena brachiocephalica)

7. **Right brachiocephalic vein** (Vena brachiocephalica)

8. **Superior vena cava** (Vena cava superior)

9. **Right superior pulmonary vein** (Vena pulmonalis)

10. **Right pulmonary artery** (Arteria pulmonalis)

11. **Right inferior lobar bronchus** (Bronchus lobaris inferior dexter)

12. **Azygos vein** (Vena azygos)

13. **Left atrium** (Atrium sinistrum)

14. **Right atrium** (Atrium dextrum)

15. **Ascending aorta** (Aorta ascendens)

16. **Right ventricle** (Ventriculus dexter)

17. **Oesophagus** (Oesophagus)

18. **Descending aorta** (Aorta descendens)

VII – Right Ventricle and Aortic Valves T – 7

In this section, the thorax has been sliced at T-7 and rotated to show structures on the left.
The lumen of the right ventricle sits posterior to the thymus, and can be traced back to the pulmonary trunk. The aorta can be followed from its orifice to its arch and descending component. The left pulmonary veins merge with the left atrium, posterior to which sit the oesophagus and azygos vein. Note the right lung, where lobar grooves separate the lung into superior, middle, and inferior lobes. A corresponding CT shows these structures radiographically.

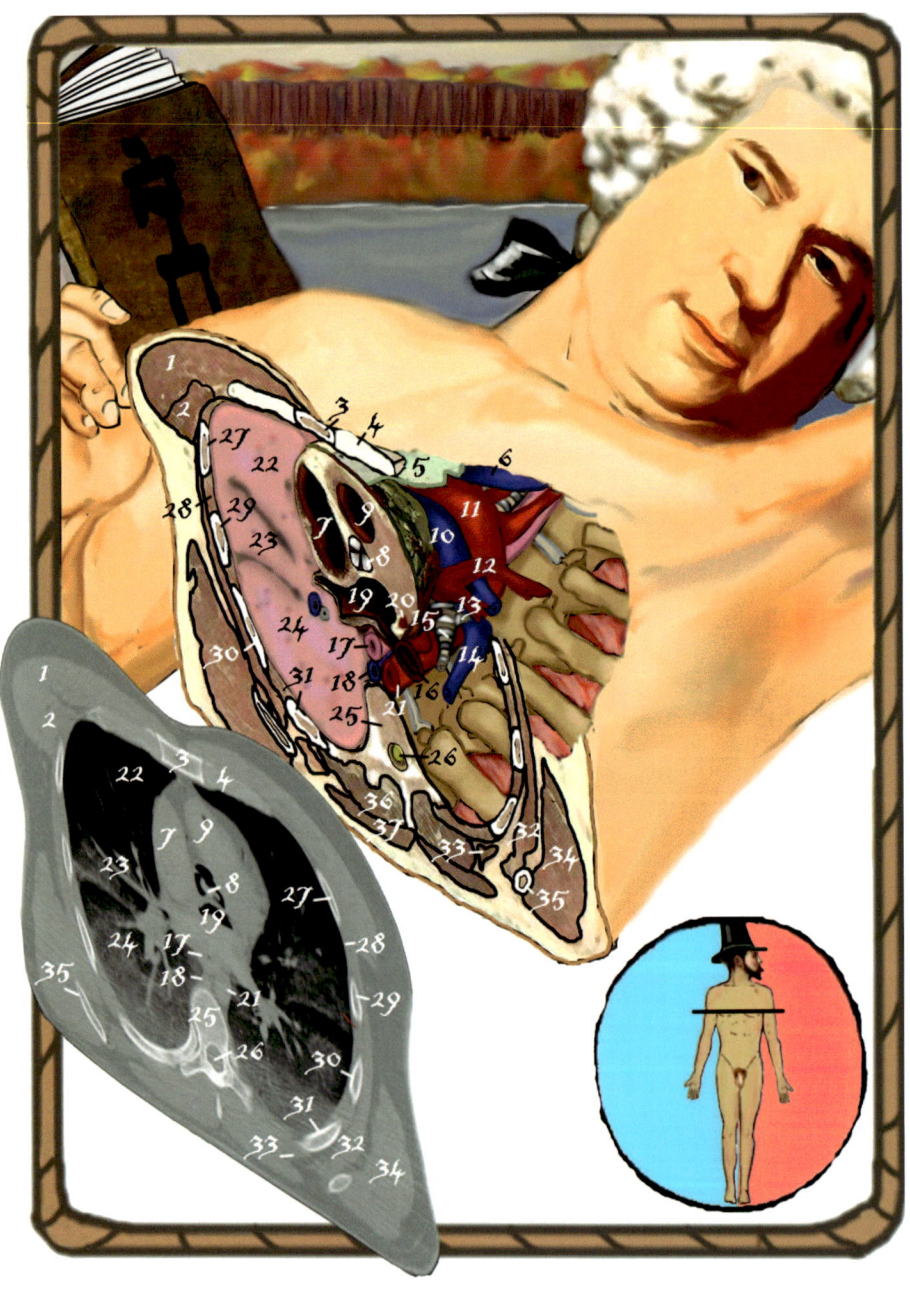

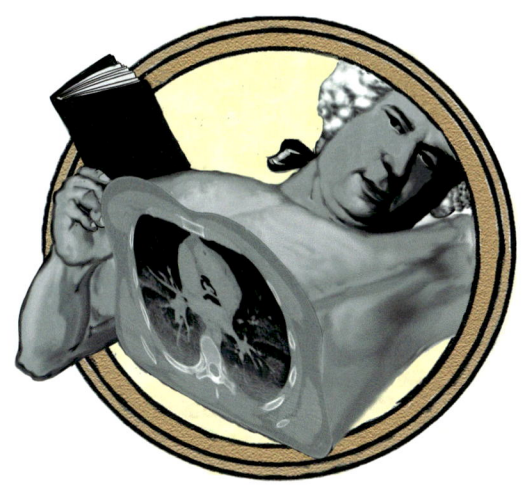

1. **Pectoralis major** (M. pectoralis major)

2. **Pectoralis minor** (M. pectoralis minor)

3. **Sternum** (Sternum)

4. **Costal cartilage of the third rib** (Cartilago costalis)

5. **Thymus** (Thymus)

6. **Left brachiocephalic vein** (Vena brachiocephalica)

7. **Right atrium** (Atrium dextrum)

8. **Aortic orifice and valve** (Ostium aortae et valva aorta)

9. **Right ventricle** (Ventriculus dexter)

10. **Pulmonary trunk** (Truncus pulmonalis)

11. **Arch of aorta** (Arcus aortae)

12. **Left superior pulmonary vein** (Vena pulmonalis)

13. **Left middle pulmonary vein** (Vena pulmonalis)

14. **Left pulmonary artery** (Arteria pulmonalis)

15. **Left inferior lobar bronchus** (Bronchus lobaris inferior sinister)

16. **Left inferior pulmonary vein** (Vena pulmonalis)

17. **Oesophagus** (Oesophagus)

18. **Azygos vein** (Vena azygos)

19. **Left atrium** (Atrium sinistrum)

20. **Left circumflex artery** (Arteria circumflexus)

21. **Descending aorta** (Aorta descendens)

22. **Superior lobe of the right lung** (Pulmo dexter, lobus superior)

23. **Middle lobe of the right lung** (Pulmo dexter, lobus medius)

24. **Inferior lobe of the right lung** (Pulmo dexter, lobus inferior)

25. **Seventh thoracic vertebra** (Vertebra thoracica septima)

26. **Spinal cord** (Medulla spinalis)

27. **Fourth rib** (Costa quarta)

28. **Intercostal muscles** (Mm. intercostales)

29. **Fifth rib** (Costa quinta)

30. **Sixth rib** (Costa sexta)

31. **Seventh rib** (Costa septima)

32. **Serratus anterior** (M. serratus anterior)

33. **Rhomboid major** (M. rhomboideus major)

34. **Latissimus dorsi** (M. Latissimus dorsi)

35. **Scapula** (Scapula)

36. **Erector spinae** (M. erector spinae)

37. **Trapezius** (M. trapezius)

VIII – Atrioventricular Valves T – 8

In this section, the thorax has been sliced at T-8 and rotated to show structures on the left. The right atrium is separated from the right ventricle by the tricuspid valve, seen in the midline. Posteriorly, the left atrium is separated from the left ventricle by the mitral valve. The oesophagus is directly posterior to the interventricular septum. A corresponding CT shows these structures radiographically.

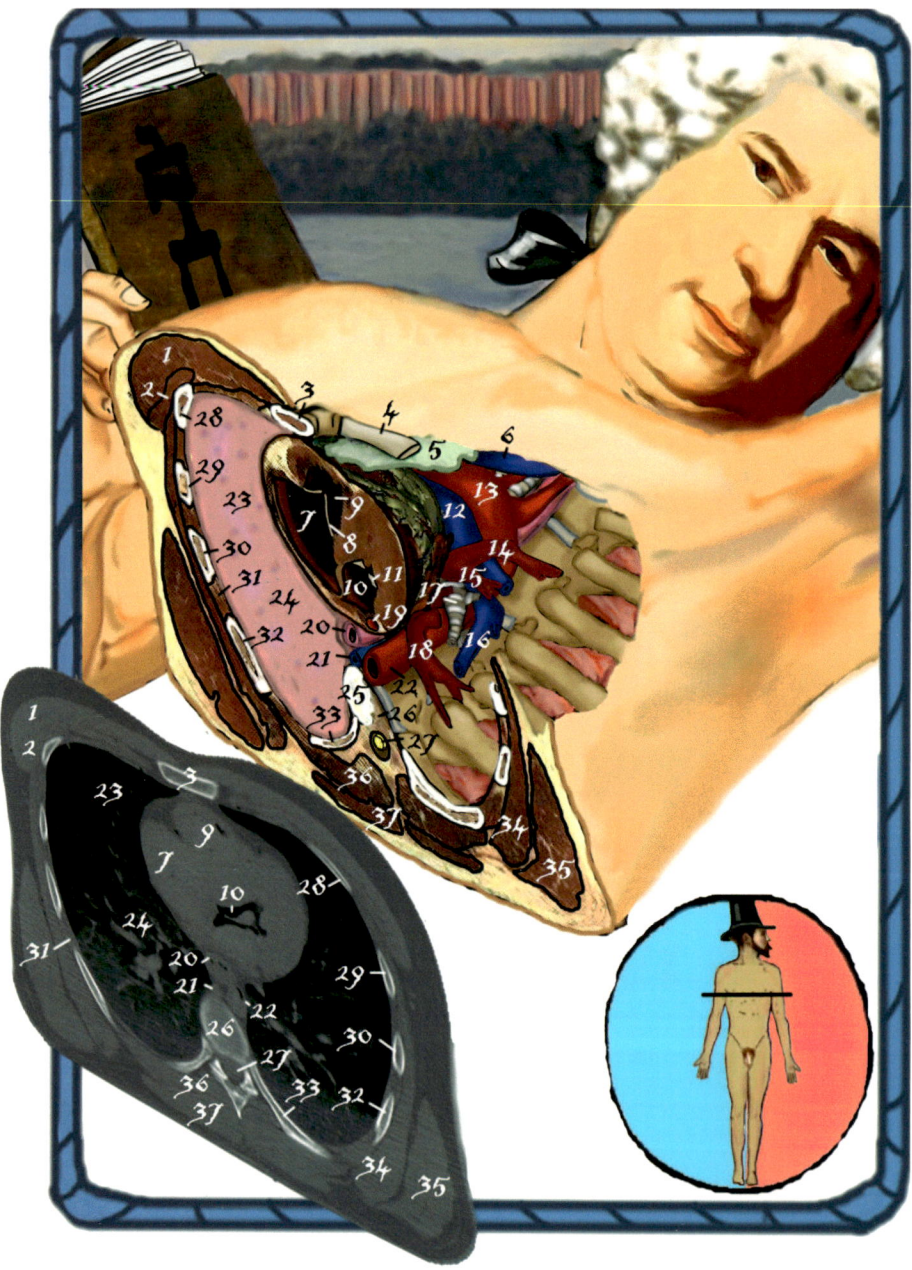

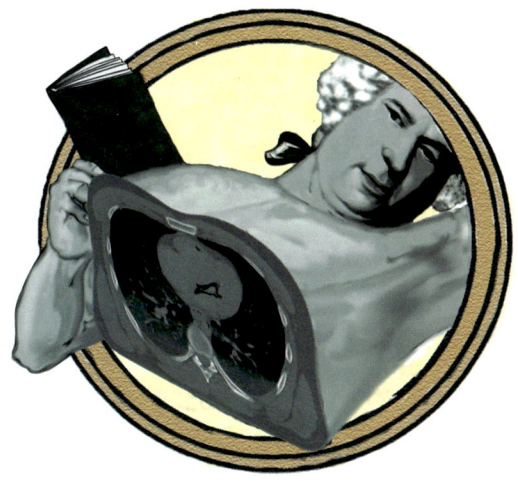

1. **Pectoralis major** (M. pectoralis major)
2. **Pectoralis minor** (M. pectoralis minor)
3. **Sternum** (Sternum)
4. **Costal cartilage of the third rib** (Cartilago costalis)
5. **Thymus** (Thymus)
6. **Left brachiocephalic vein** (Vena brachiocephalica)
7. **Right atrium** (Atrium dextrum)
8. **Tricuspid valve** (Valva atrioventricularis dextra, tricuspidalis) Derived from the Latin term for three, tres, and cuspis, a point, the valve was described by Erasistratus in the 3rd century BC.
9. **Right ventricle** (Ventriculus dexter)
10. **Left atrium** (Atrium sinister)
11. **Mitral valve** (Valva atrioventricularis sinistra, mitralis) Derived from mitre, a type of hat worn by clergy, the term was introduced to anatomy by Vesalius.
12. **Pulmonary trunk** (Truncus pulmonalis)
13. **Arch of aorta** (Arcus aortae)
14. **Left superior pulmonary vein** (Vena pulmonalis)
15. **Left middle pulmonary vein** (Vena pulmonalis)

16. **Left pulmonary artery** (Arteria pulmonalis)
17. **Left inferior lobar bronchus** (Bronchus lobaris inferior sinister)
18. **Left inferior pulmonary vein** (Vena pulmonalis)
19. **Left circumflex artery** (Arteria circumflexus)
20. **Oesophagus** (Oesophagus)
21. **Azygos vein** (Vena azygos) Derived from, άζυξ, meaning unpaired, the vein was named by Galen in the 2nd century.
22. **Descending aorta** (Aorta descendens)
23. **Superior lobe of the right lung** (Pulmo dexter, lobus superior)
24. **Inferior lobe of the right lung** (Pulmo dexter, lobus inferior)
25. **Intervertebral disc** (Discus intervertebralis)
26. **Eighth thoracic vertebra** (Vertebra thoracica octava)
27. **Spinal cord** (Medulla spinalis)
28. **Fifth rib** (Costa quinta)
29. **Sixth rib** (Costa sexta)
30. **Seventh rib** (Costa septima)
31. **Intercostal muscles** (Mm. intercostales)
32. **Eighth rib** (Costa octava)
33. **Ninth rib** (Costa nona)
34. **Serratus anterior** (M. serratus anterior)
35. **Latissimus dorsi** (M. Latissimus dorsi)
36. **Erector spinae** (M. erector spinae)
37. **Trapezius** (M. trapezius)

VIII – Atrioventricular Valves T – 8

In this section, the thorax has been sliced at T-8 and rotated to show structures on the right. The superior vena cava can be traced to the quite spacious right atrium. The right atrium is separated from the right ventricle by the tricuspid valve, seen in the midline. Posteriorly, the left atrium is separated from the left ventricle by the mitral valve. The oesophagus is directly posterior to the interventricular and interatrial septa. Note that the angle of these septa is approximately 23 degrees, the same angle of inclination as the eyes off the sagittal midline, the distal tilt of the radius bone, and the earth on its axis. A corresponding CT shows these structures radiographically.

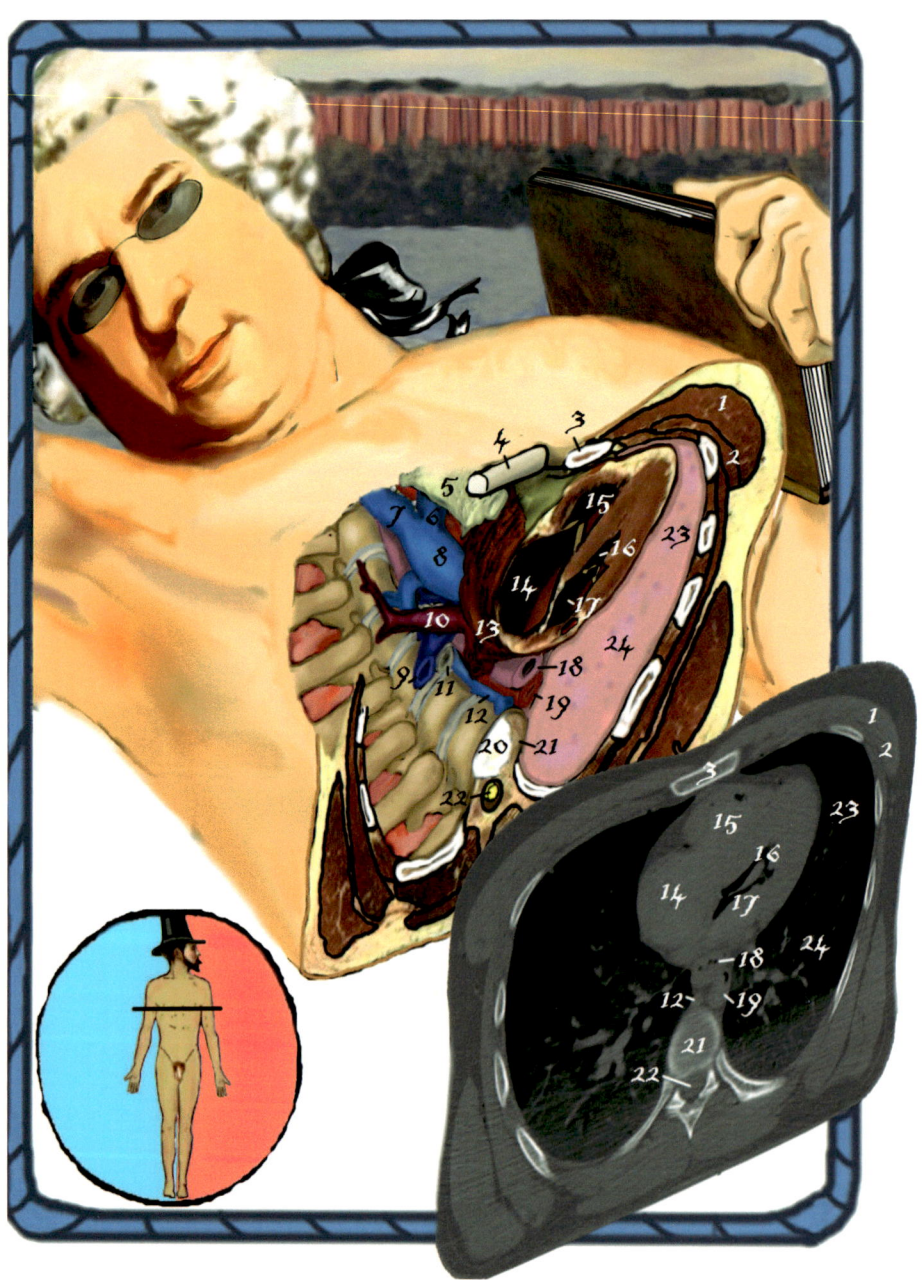

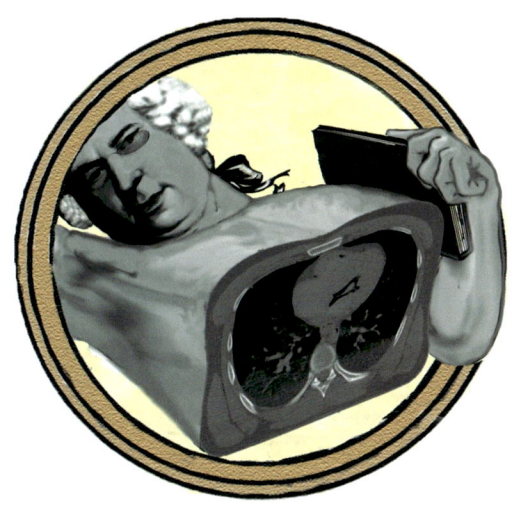

18. **Oesophagus** (Oesophagus)

19. **Descending aorta** (Aorta descendens)

20. **Intervertebral disc** (Discus intervertebralis)

21. **Eighth thoracic vertebra** (Vertebra thoracica octava)

22. **Spinal cord** (Medulla spinalis)

23. **Superior lobe of the left lung** (Pulmo sinister, lobus superior)

24. **Inferior lobe of the left lung** (Pulmo sinister, lobus inferior)

1. **Pectoralis major** (M. pectoralis major)

2. **Pectoralis minor** (M. pectoralis minor)

3. **Sternum** (Sternum)

4. **Costal cartilage of the third rib** (Cartilago costalis)

5. **Thymus** (Thymus)

6. **Left brachiocephalic vein** (Vena brachiocephalica)

7. **Right brachiocephalic vein** (Vena brachiocephalica)

8. **Superior vena cava** (Vena cava superior)

9. **Right pulmonary artery** (Arteria pulmonalis)

10. **Right superior pulmonary vein** (Vena pulmonalis)

11. **Right inferior lobar bronchus** (Bronchus lobaris inferior dexter)

12. **Azygos vein** (Vena azygos)

13. **Right middle and inferior pulmonary veins** (Vena pulmonalis)

14. **Right atrium** (Atrium dextrum)

15. **Right ventricle** (Ventriculus dexter)

16. **Left ventricle** (Ventriculus sinister)

17. **Left atrium** (Atrium sinistrum)

Part Two:
The Female Thorax

IX – The Female Breast and Ribs T – 8

In this section, the female thorax has been sliced through T-8, at the level of the nipple, and rotated to show structures on the right. The muscles overlying the right thorax have been removed in order to visualize the ribs and their curvature in relation to the cross-section. Note the right lung in the coronal plane, and the interlobar grooves separating the lung into superior, middle, and inferior lobes. As this section approaches the superior diaphragmatic surface, a portion of the dome of the liver is seen. The inferior vena cava sits medial to the liver. In the left breast, the ducts and suspensory ligaments are seen directly posterior to the nipple. The interlobar groove in the left lung is seen anteriorly. During resuscitative chest compressions, blood is ejected from the heart as it is squeezed against the vertebrae. Although not appearing radiographically, the superiormost aspect of the central tendon of the diaphragm has been illustrated on the left. A corresponding CT is provided.

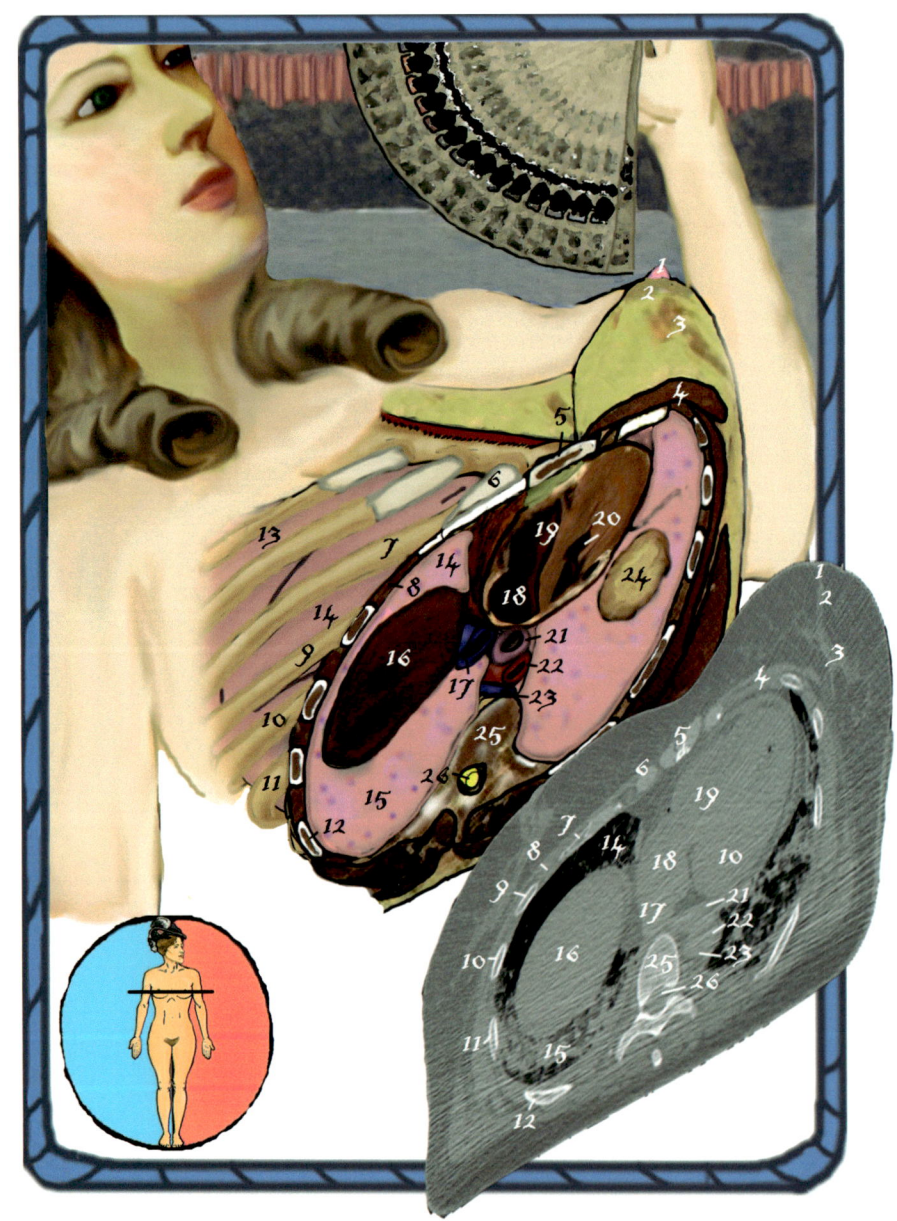

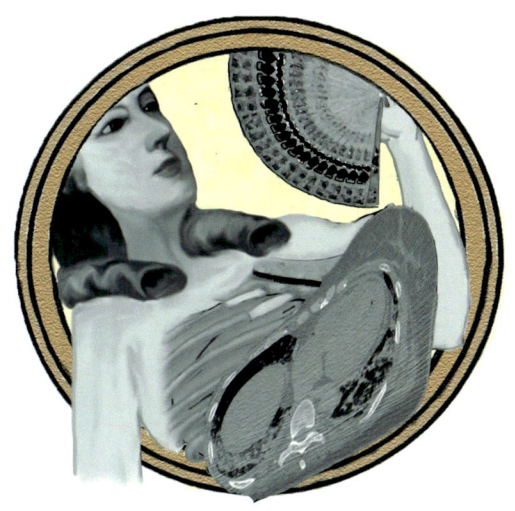

18. **Right atrium** (Atrium dextrum)

19. **Right ventricle** (Ventriculus dexter)

20. **Left ventricle** (Ventriculus sinister)

21. **Oesophagus** (Oesophagus)

22. **Descending aorta** (Aorta descendens)

23. **Azygos vein** (Vena azygos)

24. **Central tendon of the diaphragm** (Diaphragma, centrum tendineum)

25. **Eighth thoracic vertebra** (Vertebra thoracica octava)

26. **Spinal cord** (Medulla spinalis)

1. **Nipple** (Papilla mammaria)

2. **Lactiferous duct** (Ductus lactiferi)

3. **Suspensory (Cooper's) ligaments of the breast** (Lig.. suspensoria mammaria) This structure was first described by the English anatomist Astley Cooper in the 19th century.

4. **Pectoralis major** (M. pectoralis major)

5. **Sternum** (Sternum)

6. **Costal cartilage of the fourth rib** (Cartilago costalis)

7. **Fourth rib** (Costa quarta)

8. **Intercostal muscles** (Mm. intercostales)

9. **Fifth rib** (Costa quinta)

10. **Sixth rib** (Costa sexta)

11. **Seventh rib** (Costa septima)

12. **Eighth rib** (Costa octava)

13. **Superior lobe of the right lung** (Pulmo dexter, lobus superior)

14. **Middle lobe of the right lung** (Pulmo dexter, lobus medius)

15. **Inferior lobe of the right lung** (Pulmo dexter, lobus inferior)

16. **Liver** (Hepar)

17. **Inferior vena cava** (Vena cava inferior)

X – The Female Breast and Thoracic Musculature T – 8

In this section, the female thorax has been sliced through T-8, at the level of the nipple, and rotated to show structures on the left. The left breast has been removed in order to visualize the thoracic muscles—pectoralis major, serratus anterior, and latissimus dorsi—in relation to the cross-section. The dome of the liver is seen both in cross section, and also in the sagittal plane. The inferior vena cava is seen medial to the liver. In the right breast, the ducts and suspensory ligaments are seen directly posterior to the nipple. Note the relation of the heart to the overlying sternum and underlying vertebral column. During resuscitative chest compressions, blood is ejected from the heart as it is squeezed against the vertebrae. Although not appearing radiographically, the superiormost aspect of the central tendon of the diaphragm has been illustrated on the left. A corresponding CT is provided.

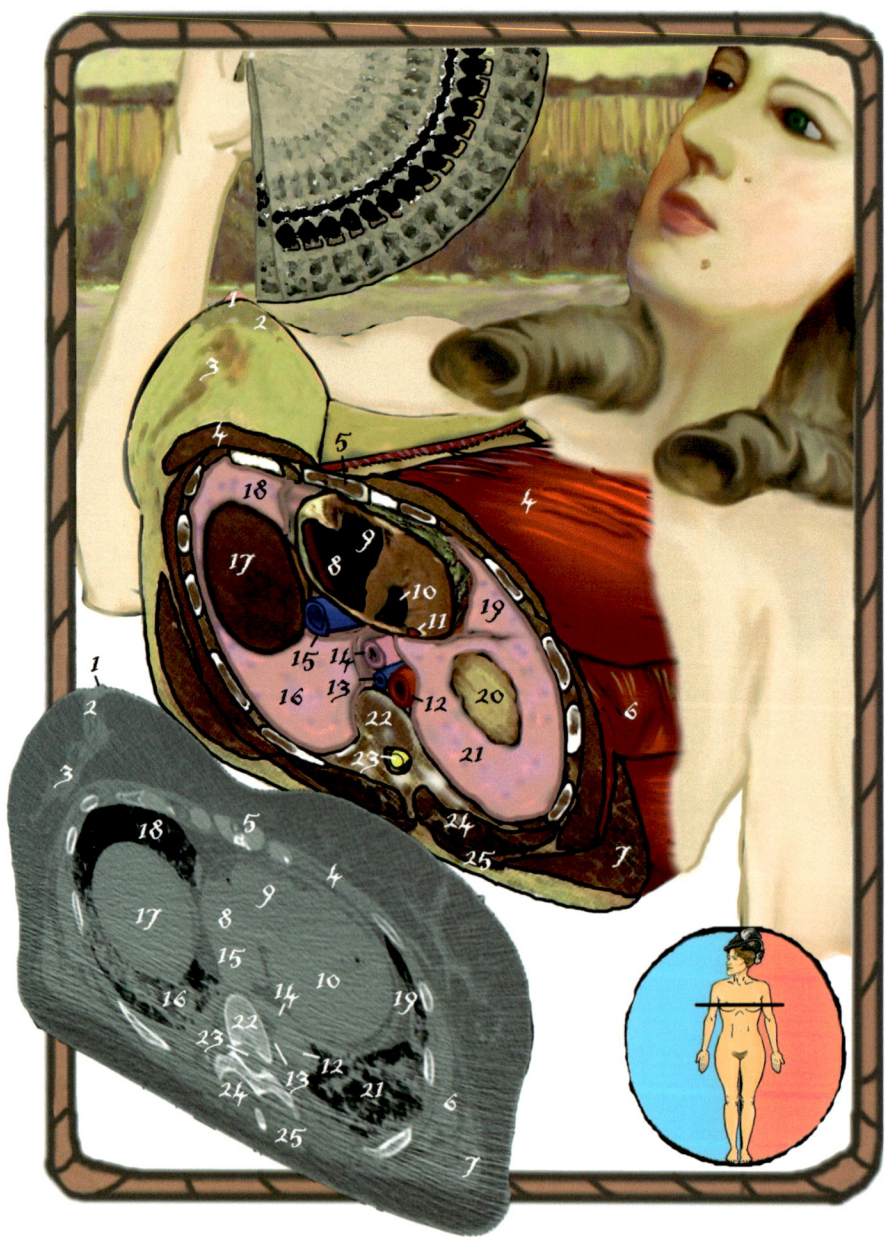

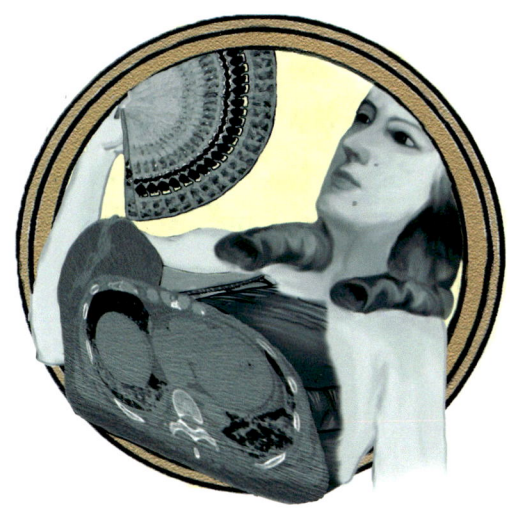

1. **Nipple** (Papilla mammaria)

2. **Lactiferous duct** (Ductus lactiferi)

3. **Suspensory (Cooper's) ligaments of the breast** (Lig. suspensoria mammaria)

4. **Pectoralis major** (M. pectoralis major)

5. **Sternum** (Sternum)

6. **Serratus anterior** (M. serratus anterior)

7. **Latissimus dorsi** (M. Latissimus dorsi)

8. **Right atrium** (Atrium dextrum)

9. **Right ventricle** (Ventriculus dexter)

10. **Left ventricle** (Ventriculus sinister)

11. **Left circumflex artery** (Arteria circumflexus)

12. **Descending aorta** (Aorta descendens)

13. **Azygos vein** (Vena azygos)

14. **Oesophagus** (Oesophagus)

15. **Inferior vena cava** (Vena cava inferior)

16. **Inferior lobe of the right lung** (Pulmo dexter, lobus inferior)

17. **Liver** (Hepar)

18. **Middle lobe of the right lung** (Pulmo dexter, lobus medius)

19. **Superior lobe of the left lung** (Pulmo sinister, lobus superior)

20. **Central tendon of the diaphragm** (Diaphragma, centrum tendineum)

21. **Inferior lobe of the left lung** (Pulmo sinister, lobus inferior)

22. **Eighth thoracic vertebra** (Vertebra thoracica octava)

23. **Spinal cord** (Medulla spinalis)

24. **Erector spinae** (M.erector spinae)

25. **Trapezius** (M. trapezius)

CHAPTER THREE
THE ABDOMEN

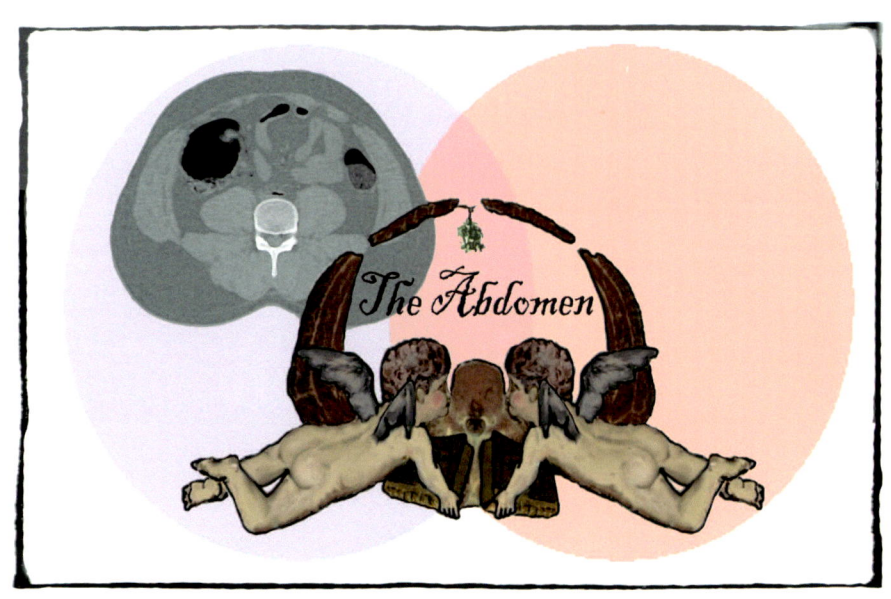

I – The Esophageal Hiatus, T – 10

According to Skinner, the term abdomen is likely derived from the Latin verb abdere, meaning to hide, as the viscera are hidden within the abdominal cavity. In this section, the abdomen has been sliced at the level of the tenth thoracic vertebra and rotated slightly to the left. The origins of rectus abdominis flank the midline, near the sternum. Just posterior to this is a pocket of thoracic fat in which sits the pericardial reflection. Serratus anterior, on the lateral abdominal wall, is tapering off at its distal insertion. The diaphragm cordons off the abdominal contents, and in the posterior midline, just superior to the vertebral body, a hiatus allows the oesophagus passage from the thorax. A corresponding CT shows these structures radiographically.

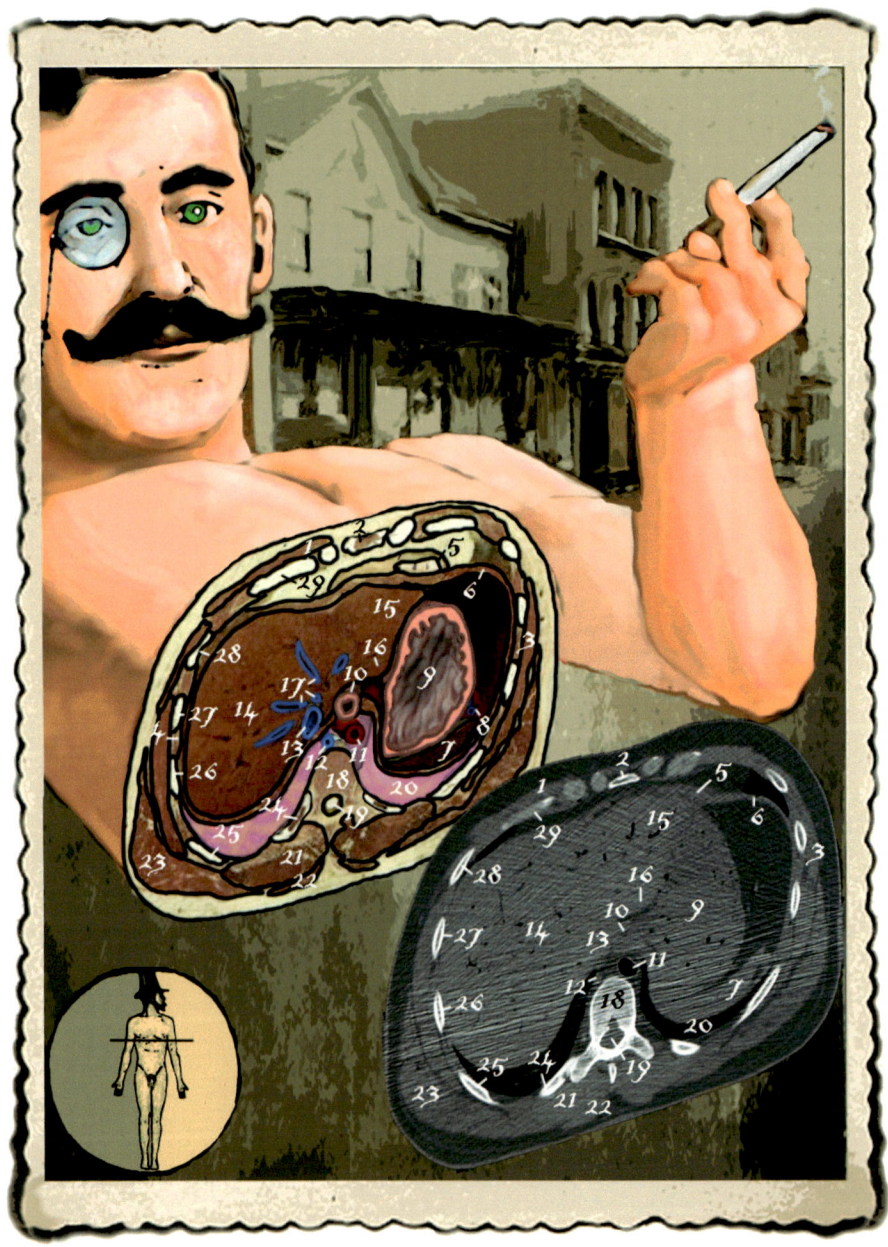

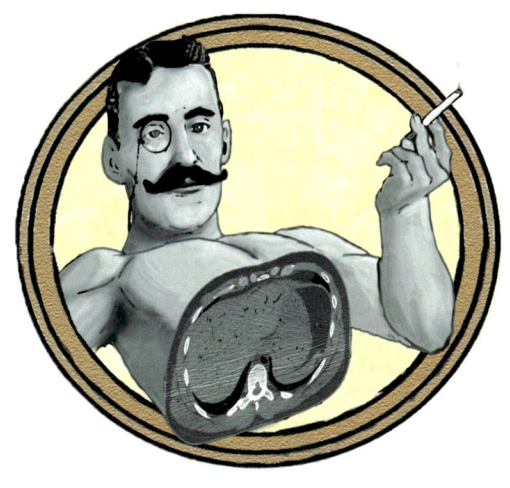

16. **Caudate lobe** (*Lobus caudatus*) Derived from the Latin cauda or coda meaning tail.

17. **Hepatic vein** (*V. hepatica*)

18. **Tenth thoracic vertebra** (*Vertebra thoracica decima*)

19. **Spinal cord** (*Medulla spinalis*)

20. **Inferior lobe of the lung** (*Pulmo, lobus inferior*)

21. **Erector spinae** (*M. erector spinae*)

22. **Trapezius** (*M. trapezius*)

23. **Latissimus dorsi** (*M. latissimus dorsi*)

24. **Tenth rib** (*Costa decima*)

25. **Ninth rib** (*Costa nona*)

26. **Eighth rib** (*Costa octava*)

27. **Seventh rib** (*Costa septima*)

28. **Sixth rib** (*Costa sexta*)

29. **Costal cartilage** (*Cartilago costalis*)

1. **Rectus Abdominis** (*M. rectus abdominis*)

2. **Sternum** (*Sternum*)

3. **Serratus anterior** (*M. serratus anterior*)

4. **Intercostal muscles** (*Mm. intercostales*)

5. **Pericardium** (*Pericardium*)

6. **Diaphragm** (*Diaphragma*) Derived from διάφραγμα, meaning a partition, the diaphragm was first named by Galen.

7. **Spleen** (*Splen/lien*)

8. **Gastro-omental artery and vein** (*A. et v. gastroomentalis*)

9. **Fundus of the stomach** (*Fundus gastricus*) Whereas the term gastric is derived from γαστηρ, meaning stomach, the term stomach is derived from στόμα, meaning mouth.

10. **Oesophagus** (*Oesophagus*)

11. **Descending aorta** (*Aorta descendens*)

12. **Azygos vein** (*Vena azygos*)

13. **Inferior vena cava** (*Vena cava inferior*)

14. **Right lobe of liver** (*Lobus hepatis dexter*) The term liver is of Anglo-Saxon origin, and the organ was believed by early anatomists to be the site of blood formation.

15. **Left lobe of liver** (*Lobus hepatis sinister*)

II – The Gastric Fundus – T-10

In this section the abdomen has been sectioned at the most inferior aspect of T – 10, and rotated slightly to the left. Just anterior to the vertebral body, the diaphragm gently wraps around the distal end of the oesophagus, as it unites with the gastric cardia. The gastric fundus curves like a slender vase. Posterior to the stomach is the spleen and the gastro-omental vessels, branches of the splenic artery and vein. The small intestines have been removed from the vivisection to better visualize the abdominal contents, however, their position can be appreciated in the corresponding CT.

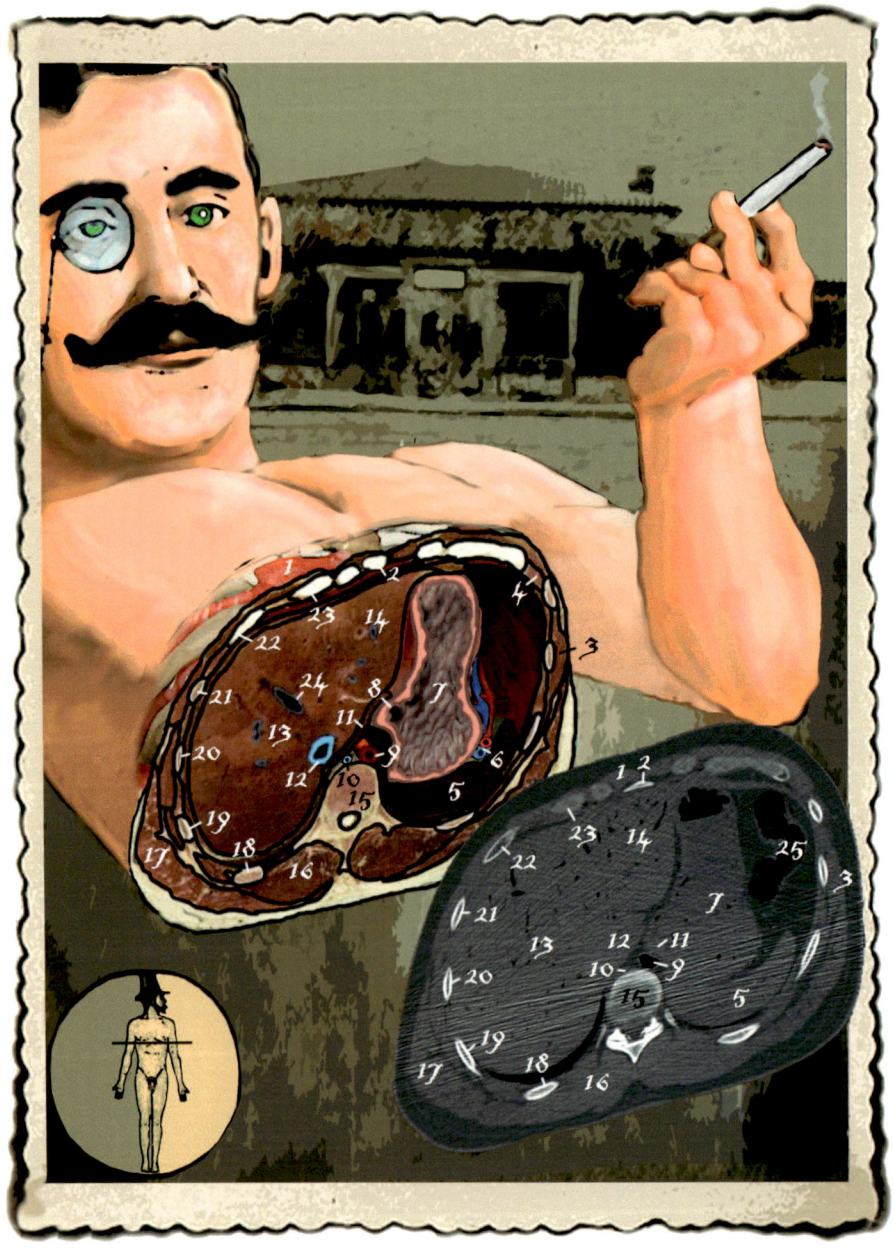

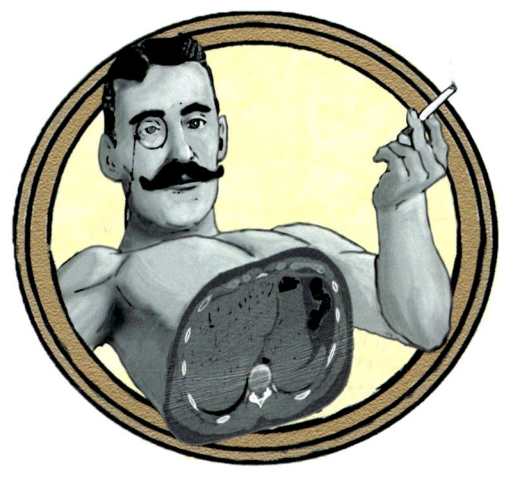

18. **Tenth rib** (*Costa decima*)

19. **Ninth rib** (*Costa nona*)

20. **Eighth rib** (*Costa octava*)

21. **Seventh rib** (*Costa septima*)

22. **Sixth rib** (*Costa sexta*)

23. **Costal cartilage** (*Cartilago costalis*)

24. **Hepatic vein** (*V. hepatica*)

25. **Jejunum** (*Jejunum*) Derived from the Latin term jejunus, which means both hungry and breakfast, the jejunum was so named by Galen as it was often found empty in dissections.

1. **Rectus Abdominis** (*M. rectus abdominis*)

2. **Xiphoid process** (*Processus xiphoideus*) Derived from, ξιφος, meaning sword, the bone was so named by Aristotle.

3. **Serratus anterior** (*M. serratus anterior*)

4. **Intercostal muscles** (*Mm. intercostales*)

5. **Spleen** (*Splen/lien*) Derived from σπλήν, the spleen was so named by Hippocrates. As Skinner points out, lien is the Latinization of the Greek, minus the "sp.'

6. **Gastro-omental artery and vein** (*A. et v. gastroomentalis*)

7. **Body of the stomach** (*Corpus gastricum*)

8. **Oesophagus** (*Oesophagus*)

9. **Descending aorta** (*Aorta descendens*)

10. **Azygos vein** (*Vena azygos*)

11. **Crus of the diaphragm** (*Crus diaphragma*)

12. **Inferior vena cava** (*Vena cava inferior*)

13. **Right lobe of liver** (*Lobus hepatis dexter*)

14. **Left lobe of liver** (*Lobus hepatis sinister*)

15. **Tenth thoracic vertebra** (*Vertebra thoracica decima*)

16. **Erector spinae** (*M. erector spinae*)

17. **Latissimus dorsi** (*M. latissimus dorsi*)

III – *Superior Duodenum, Choledochal Structures, and the Portal Triad – T- 11*

In this section, the abdomen has been sliced at the level of the eleventh thoracic vertebra and rotated slightly to the left. The pyloric antrum of the stomach makes way to the superior part of the pylorus and duodenum. In the liver, note the crescent shaped fossa formed from the left lobe supero-medially near the stomach, the concave right lobe laterally, and the caudate lobe—between the portal vein and inferior vena-cava—posteriorly. Within this space, the superior-most aspect of the hepatic flexure is flanked by the gallbladder laterally and the superior duodenum, medially. Postero-medially is the portal triad, composed of the hepatic duct, the portal vein, and the left hepatic artery. The cystic duct and right hepatic artery are more lateral. The small intestines have been removed from the vivisection to better visualize the abdominal contents, however, their position can be appreciated in the corresponding CT.

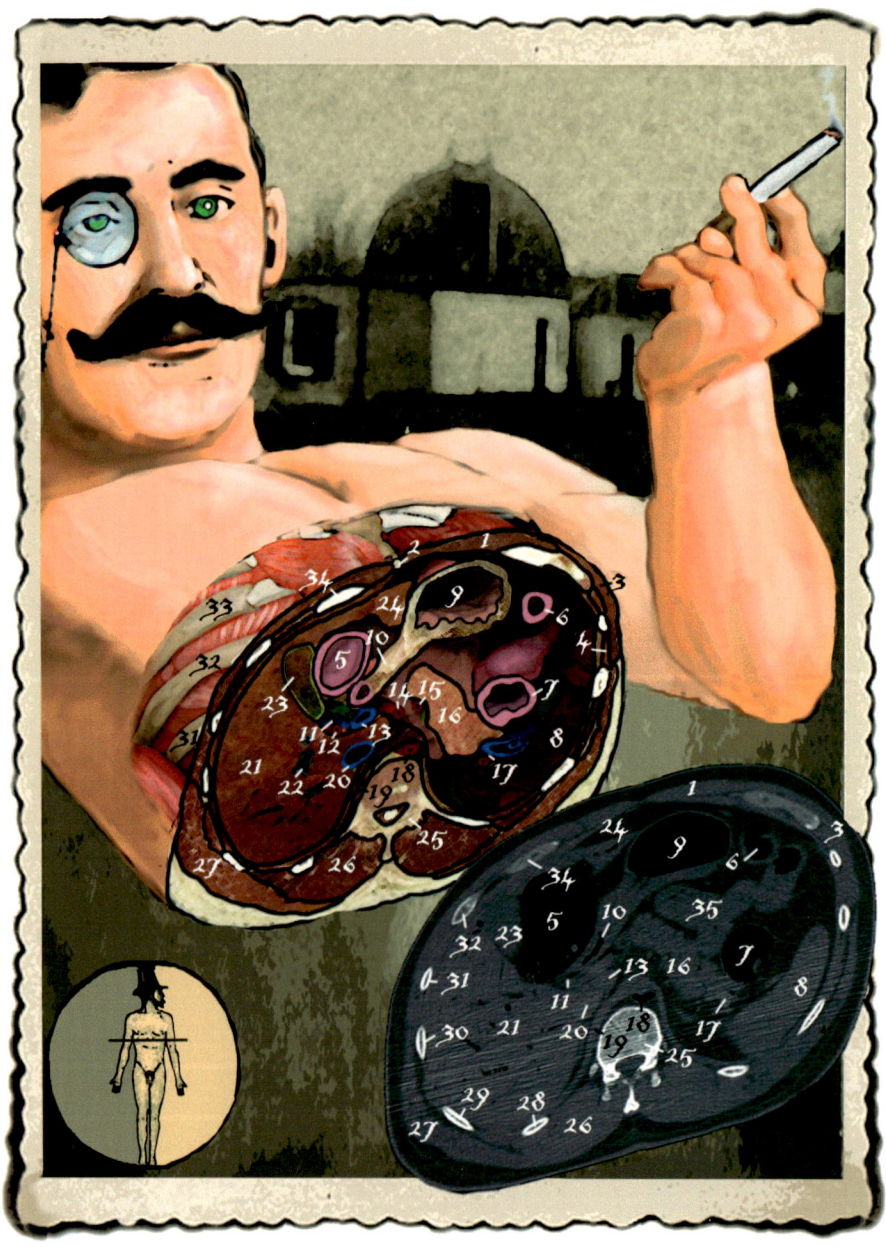

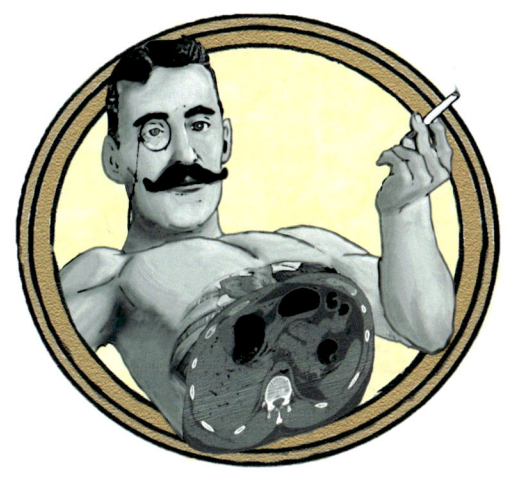

1. **Rectus Abdominis** (*M. rectus abdominis*)

2. **Xiphoid process** (*Processus xiphoideus*)

3. **External oblique** (*M. obliquus externus abdominis*)

4. **Intercostal muscles** (*Mm. intercostales*)

5. **Hepatic flexure of the colon** (*Flexura coli dextra/hepatica*)

6. **Transverse colon** (*Colon transversum*) Derived from κόλον, meaning food, the colon was so named by Aristotle.

7. **Left/splenic flexure of the colon** (*Flexura coli sinistra/splenica*)

8. **Spleen** (*Splen/lien*)

9. **Pyloric antrum** (*Antrum pyloricum*)

10. **Pylorus and superior part of the duodenum** (*Pylorus et duodenum pars superior*) Derived from πυλωρός, meaning gatekeeper, the Pylorus was so named by Celsus.

11. **Cystic and common hepatic ducts** (*Ductus cysticus et ductus hepaticus communis*)

12. **Right hepatic artery** (*A. hepatica, r. dexter*)

13. **Portal vein** (*Vena portae hepatis*)

14. **Left hepatic artery** (*A. hepatica, r. sinister*)

15. **Left gastric artery** (*A. gastrica sinistra*)

16. **Tail of the pancreas** (*Cauda pancreatis*)

17. **Splenic artery and vein** (*A. et v. splenica/linealis*)

18. **Descending aorta** (*Aorta descendens*)

19. **Crus of the diaphragm** (*Crus diaphragma*)

20. **Inferior vena cava** (*Vena cava inferior*)

21. **Right lobe of liver** (*Lobus hepatis dexter*)

22. **Hepatic vein** (*V. hepatica*)

23. **Body of the gallbladder** (*Corpus vesicae billaris/fellea*)

24. **Left lobe of liver** (*Lobus hepatis sinister*)

25. **Eleventh thoracic vertebra** (*Vertebra thoracica undecima*)

26. **Erector spinae** (*M. erector spinae*)

27. **Latissimus dorsi** (*M. latissimus dorsi*)

28. **Eleventh rib** (*Costa undecima*)

29. **Tenth rib** (*Costa decima*)

30. **Ninth rib** (*Costa nona*)

31. **Eighth rib** (*Costa octava*)

32. **Seventh rib** (*Costa septima*)

33. **Sixth rib** (*Costa sexta*)

34. **Costal cartilage** (*Cartilago costalis*)

35. **Jejunum** (*Jejunum*)

IV – The Aortic Hiatus and Pyloric Sphincter – T – 12

In this section, the abdomen has been sliced at the inferior aspect of the twelfth thoracic vertebra and rotated slightly to the left. The pyloric antrum of the stomach is slightly left of the midline, posterior to rectus abdominis and the left lobe of the liver. The pyloric sphincter runs obliquely from about 1 o'clock down to the opening of the superior part of the duodenum at about 8 o'clock. In the midline, just superior to the vertebral body, a slight hiatus allows passage of the descending aorta into the abdominal cavity, where it becomes the abdominal aorta. The left suprarenal gland sits above the superior-most aspect of the left kidney. The small intestines have been removed from the vivisection to better visualize the abdominal contents, however, their position can be appreciated in the corresponding CT.

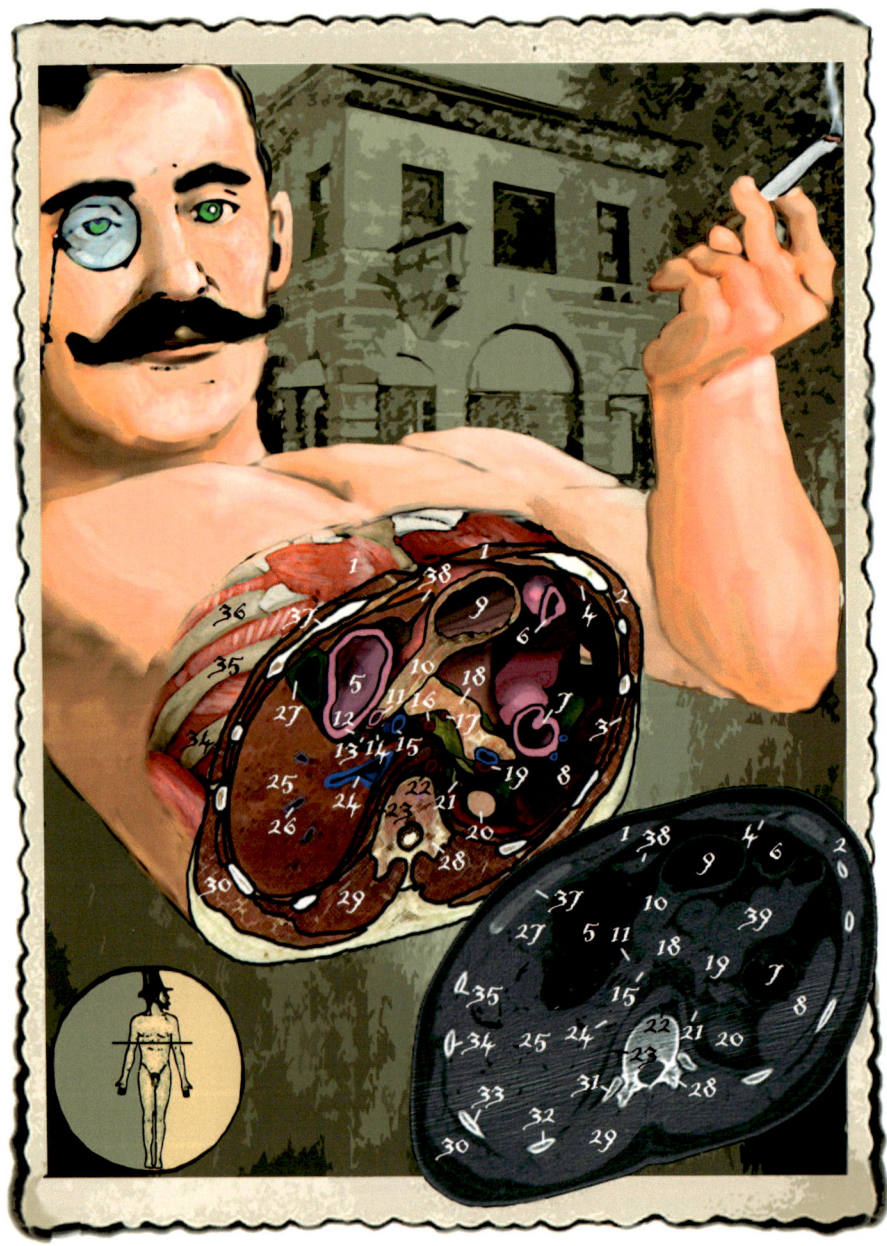

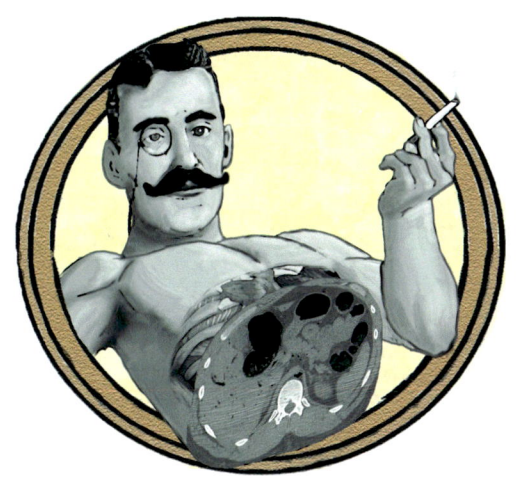

17. **Left gastric artery** (*A. gastrica sinistra*)

18. **Body of the pancreas** (*Corpus pancreatis*) Derived from πάγκρεας, meaning sweetbread, the pancreas was so named by Herophilus.

19. **Splenic artery and vein** (*A. et v. splenica/linealis*)

20. **Kidney** (*Ren/nephros*)

21. **Suprarenal gland** (*Glandula suprarenalis*) Derived from the Latin supra, or above, and ren, meaning kidney, the suprarenal glands were first described by Eustachius.

22. **Abdominal aorta** (*Aorta abdominalis*)

23. **Crus of the diaphragm** (*Crus diaphragma*)

24. **Inferior vena cava** (*Vena cava inferior*)

25. **Right lobe of liver** (*Lobus hepatis dexter*)

26. **Hepatic vein** (*V. hepatica*)

27. **Body of the gallbladder** (*Corpus vesicae billaris/fellea*)

28. **Twelfth thoracic vertebra** (*Vertebra thoracica duodecima*)

29. **Erector spinae** (*M. erector spinae*)

30. **Latissimus dorsi** (*M. latissimus dorsi*)

31. **Eleventh rib** (*Costa undecima*)

32. **Tenth rib** (*Costa decima*)

33. **Ninth rib** (*Costa nona*)

34. **Eighth rib** (*Costa octava*)

35. **Seventh rib** (*Costa septima*)

36. **Sixth rib** (*Costa sexta*)

37. **Costal cartilage** (*Cartilago costalis*)

38. **Left lobe of liver** (*Lobus hepatis sinister*)

39. **Jejunum** (*Jejunum*)

1. **Rectus Abdominis** (*M. rectus abdominis*)

2. **External oblique** (*M. obliquus externus abdominis*)

3. **Intercostal muscles** (*Mm. intercostales*)

4. **Transversus abdominis** (*M. transversus abdominis*)

5. **Hepatic flexure of the colon** (*Flexura coli dextra/hepatica*)

6. **Transverse colon** (*Colon transversum*)

7. **Left/splenic flexure of the colon** (*Flexura coli sinistra/splenica*)

8. **Spleen** (*Splen/lien*)

9. **Pyloric antrum** (*Antrum pyloricum*)

10. **Pyloric sphincter** (*M. sphincter pyloricus*)

11. **Superior part of the duodenum** (*Duodenum pars descendens*) Derived from the Latin, duodecima, meaning twelve, the duodenum was so named by Herophilus as it was about 12 fingerbreadths in length.

12. **Cystic duct** (*Ductus cysticus*)

13. **Right hepatic artery** (*A. hepatica, r. dexter*)

14. **Common hepatic duct** (*Ductus hepaticus communis*)

15. **Portal vein** (*Vena portae hepatis*)

16. **Left hepatic artery** (*A. hepatica, r. sinister*)

V – The Aortic Hiatus and the Suprarenal Glands – T – 12

In this section, the abdomen has been sliced at the inferior aspect of the twelfth thoracic vertebra and rotated slightly to the left. Posterior to the pyloric antrum and the inferior-most aspect of the pylorus is the body of the pancreas. The bile duct is to the left, while the portal vein, common hepatic artery, and left gastric artery are posterior. The aorta and aortic hiatus is seen in the midline just anterior to the vertebral body, a structure that is flanked by the left and right suprarenal glands. The small intestines have been removed from the vivisection to better visualize the abdominal contents, however, their position can be appreciated in the corresponding CT.

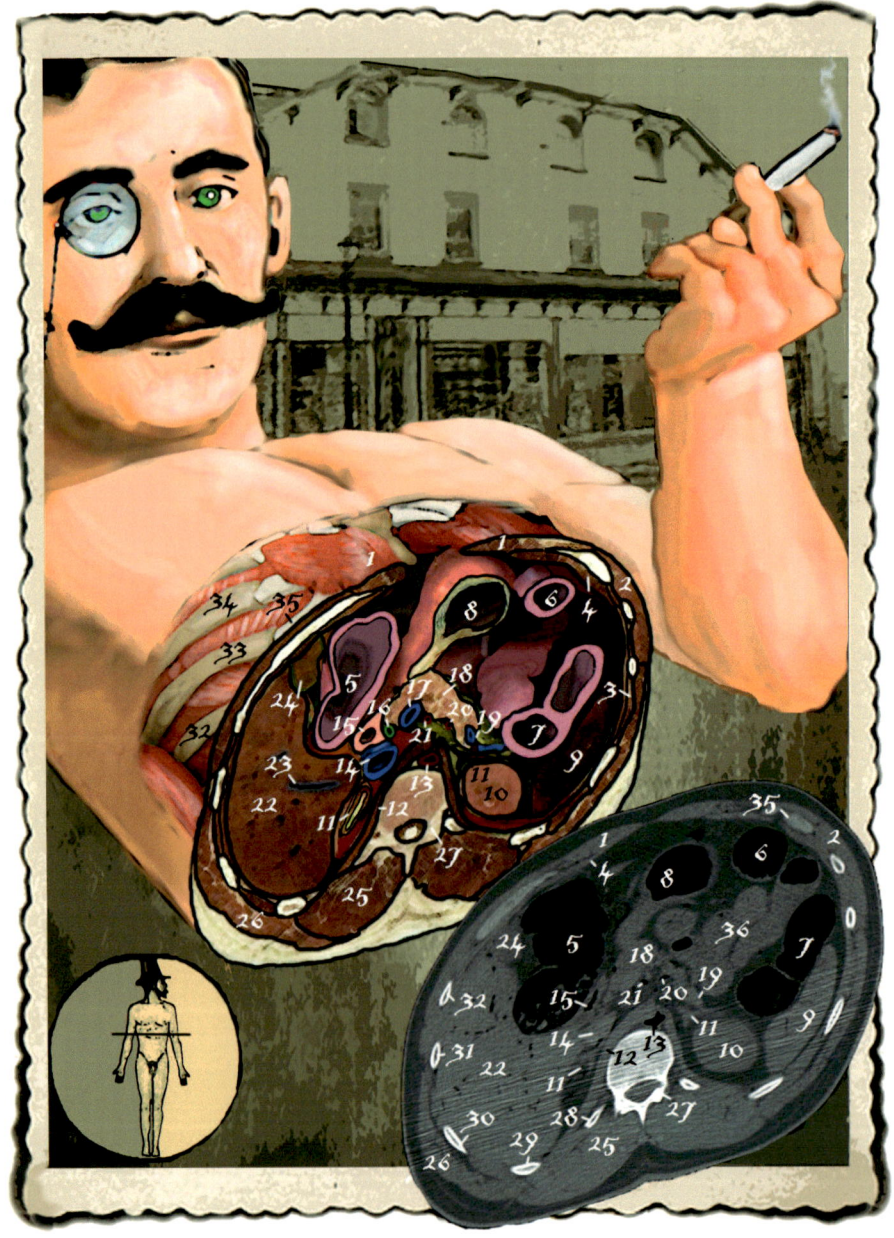

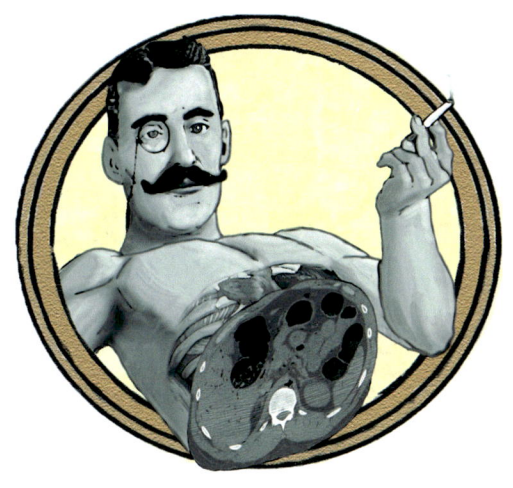

1. **Rectus Abdominis** (*M. rectus abdominis*)

2. **External oblique** (*M. obliquus externus abdominis*)

3. **Intercostal muscles** (*Mm. intercostales*)

4. **Transversus abdominis** (*M. transversus abdominis*)

5. **Hepatic flexure of the colon** (*Flexura coli dextra/hepatica*)

6. **Transverse colon** (*Colon transversum*)

7. **Left/splenic flexure of the colon** (*Flexura coli sinistra/splenica*)

8. **Pyloric antrum** (*Antrum pyloricum*)

9. **Spleen** (*Splen/lien*)

10. **Kidney** (*Ren/nephros*)

11. **Suprarenal gland** (*Glandula suprarenalis*)

12. **Crus of the diaphragm** (*Crus diaphragma*)

13. **Abdominal aorta** (*Aorta abdominalis*)

14. **Inferior vena cava** (*Vena cava inferior*)

15. **Descending part of the duodenum** (*Duodenum pars descendens*)

16. **Bile duct** (*Ductus choledochus/biliaris*)

17. **Portal vein** (*Vena portae hepatis*)

18. **Body of the pancreas** (*Corpus pancreatis*)

19. **Splenic vein and artery** (*V. et a. splenica/linealis*)

20. **Left gastric artery** (*A. gastrica sinistra*)

21. **Common hepatic artery** (*A. hepatica communis*)

22. **Right lobe of liver** (*Lobus hepatis dexter*)

23. **Hepatic vein** (*V. hepatica*)

24. **Body of the gallbladder** (*Corpus vesicae billaris/fellea*)

25. **Erector spinae** (*M. erector spinae*)

26. **Latissimus dorsi** (*M. latissimus dorsi*)

27. **Twelfth thoracic vertebra** (*Vertebra thoracica duodecima*)

28. **Twelfth rib** (*Costa duodecima*)

29. **Eleventh rib** (*Costa undecima*)

30. **Tenth rib** (*Costa decima*)

31. **Ninth rib** (*Costa nona*)

32. **Eighth rib** (*Costa octava*)

33. **Seventh rib** (*Costa septima*)

34. **Sixth rib** (*Costa sexta*)

35. **Costal cartilage** (*Cartilago costalis*)

36. **Jejunum** (*Jejunum*)

VI – Union of the Superior Mesenteric and Splenic Veins and the Coeliac Trunk – T-12/L-1

In this section, the abdomen has been sliced through the intervertebral disc between the twelfth thoracic and first lumbar vertebrae and rotated slightly to the left. The antrum of the stomach and pylorus occupy a position near the midline, posterior to rectus abdominis. The descending duodenum sits lateral to the bile duct, now thoroughly ensconced within the head of the pancreas. The superior mesenteric vein has merged with the splenic vein to form the portal vein. Posterior to this is the coeliac trunk giving rise to the splenic, hepatic, and left gastric arteries. The left suprarenal gland may be seen to the left of the vertebral body, superior to the superior pole of the left kidney. Posterior to the inferior vena cava is the right suprarenal gland. Both the hepatic and splenic flexures of the colon are clearly visible. The small intestines have been removed from the vivisection to better visualize the abdominal contents, however, their position can be appreciated in the corresponding CT.

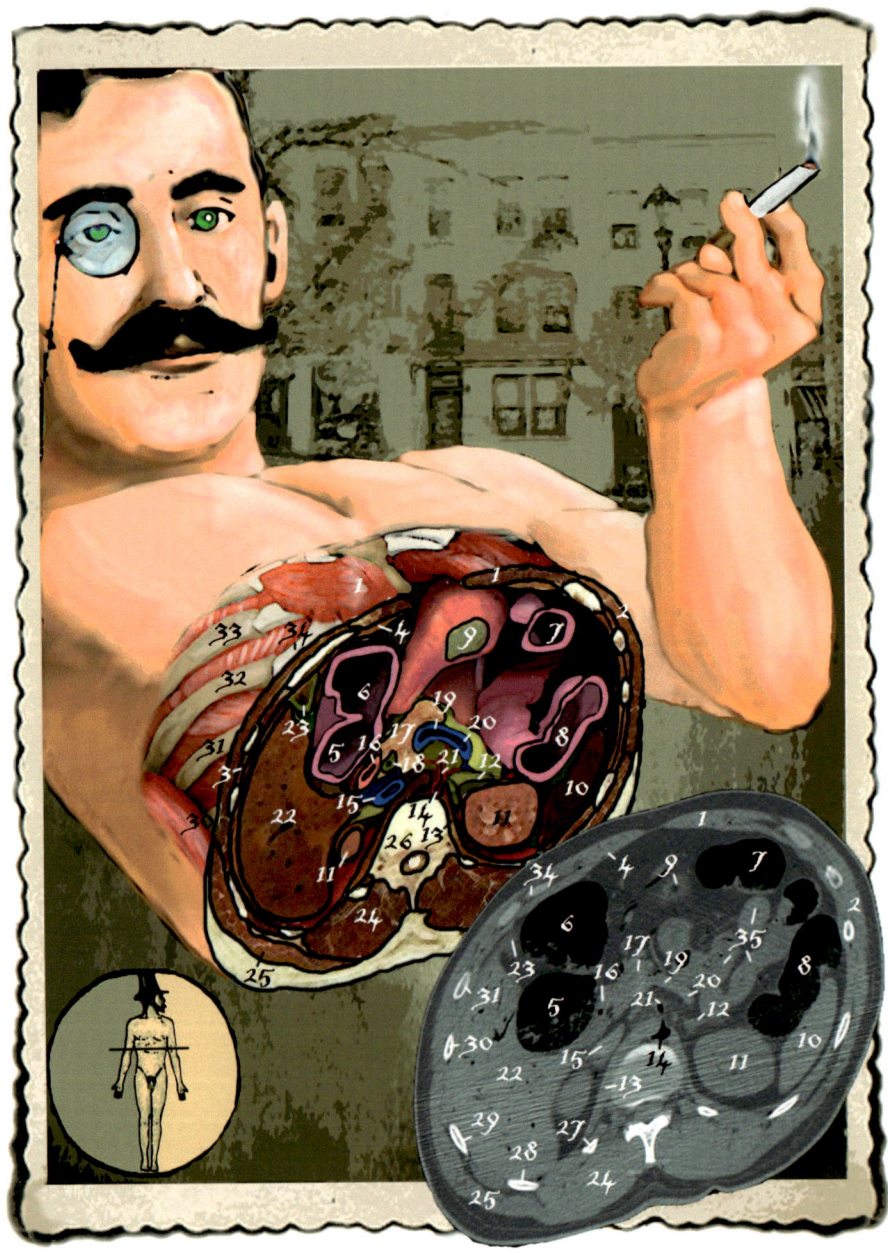

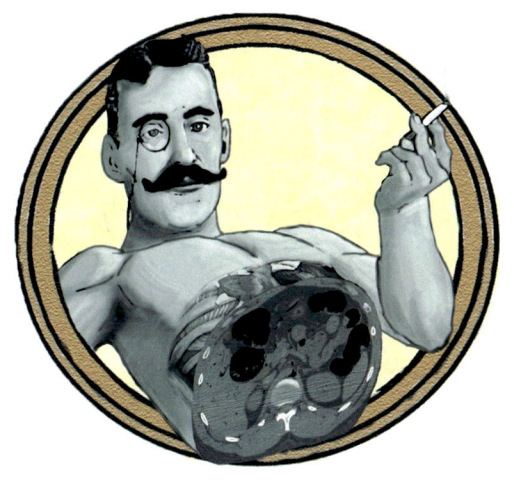

19. **Union of the superior mesenteric and splenic veins to form the portal vein** (*Vena portae hepatis*)

20. **Splenic vein** (*V. splenica/linealis*)

21. **Coeliac trunk** (*Truncus coeliacus*)

22. **Right lobe of liver** (*Lobus hepatis dexter*)

23. **Body of the gallbladder** (*Corpus vesicae billaris/fellea*)

24. **Erector spinae** (*M. erector spinae*)

25. **Latissimus dorsi** (*M. latissimus dorsi*)

26. **Intervertebral disc between T-12 and L-1** (*Discus intervertebralis*)

27. **Twelfth rib** (*Costa duodecima*)

28. **Eleventh rib** (*Costa undecima*)

29. **Tenth rib** (*Costa decima*)

30. **Ninth rib** (*Costa nona*)

31. **Eighth rib** (*Costa octava*)

32. **Seventh rib** (*Costa septima*)

33. **Sixth rib** (*Costa sexta*)

34. **Costal cartilage** (*Cartilago costalis*)

35. **Jejunum** (*Jejunum*)

1. **Rectus Abdominis** (*M. rectus abdominis*)

2. **External oblique** (*M. obliquus externus abdominis*)

3. **Intercostal muscles** (*Mm. intercostales*)

4. **Transversus abdominis** (*M. transversus abdominis*)

5. **Ascending colon** (*Colon ascendens*)

6. **Hepatic flexure of the colon** (*Flexura coli dextra/hepatica*)

7. **Transverse colon** (*Colon transversum*)

8. **Left/splenic flexure of the colon** (*Flexura coli sinistra/splenica*)

9. **Pyloric antrum** (*Antrum pyloricum*)

10. **Spleen** (*Splen/lien*)

11. **Kidney** (*Ren/nephros*)

12. **Suprarenal gland** (*Glandula suprarenalis*)

13. **Crus of the diaphragm** (*Crus diaphragma*)

14. **Abdominal aorta** (*Aorta abdominalis*)

15. **Inferior vena cava** (*Vena cava inferior*)

16. **Descending part of the duodenum** (*Duodenum pars descendens*)

17. **Head of the pancreas** (*Caput pancreatis*)

18. **Bile duct** (*Ductus choledochus/biliaris*)

VII – Superior Mesenteric Artery and the Diaphragmatic Crus – L -1

In this section, the abdomen has been sliced at the level of the first lumbar vertebra and rotated slightly to the left. The body of the stomach can be seen as it tapers off into the pyloric antrum and then curves into the pylorus and duodenum. The duodenum descends lateral to the head of the pancreas. The right diaphragmatic crus may be appreciated on the left side of the superior aspect of the vertebral body. Around the midline, anterior to the vertebra, the superior mesenteric artery shoots up from the abdominal aorta. The small intestines have been removed from the vivisection to better visualize the abdominal contents, however, their position can be appreciated in the corresponding CT.

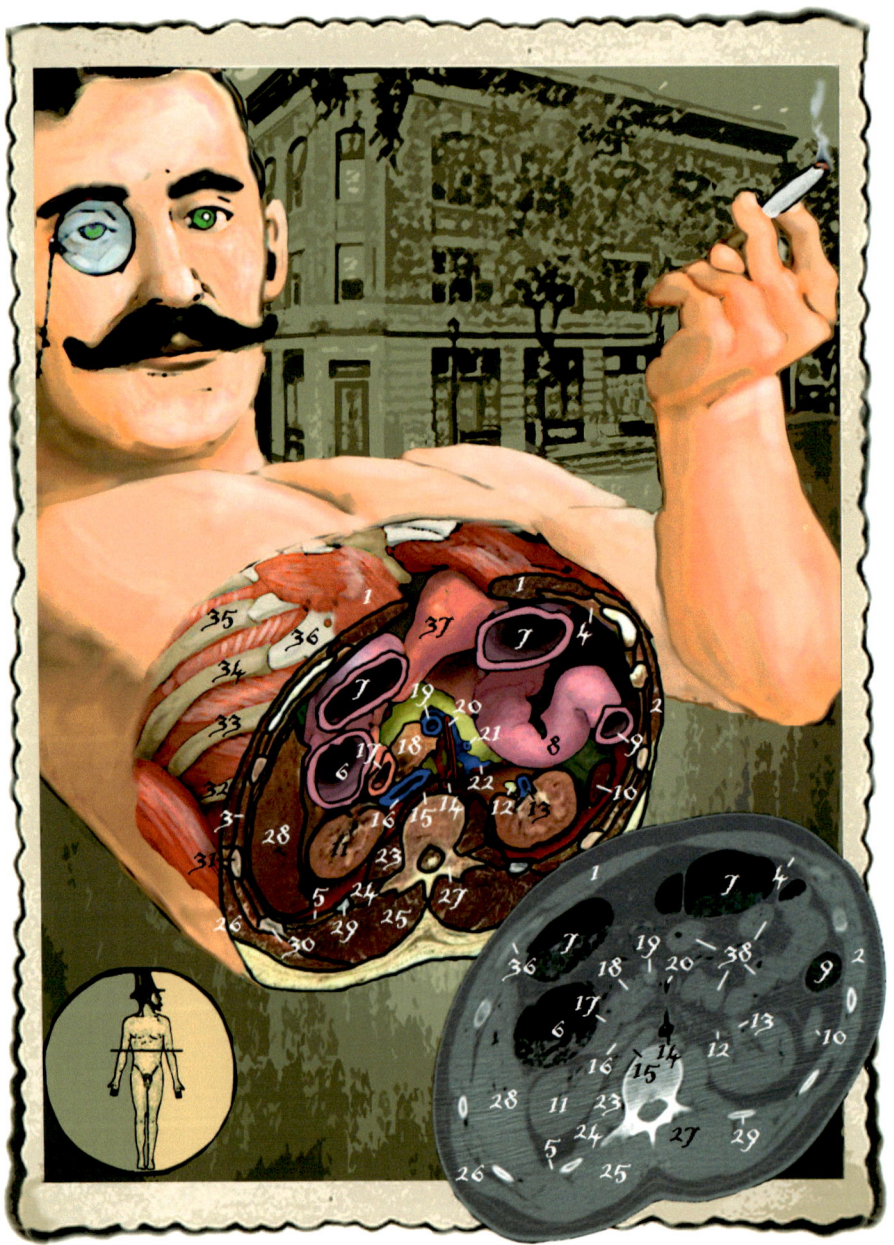

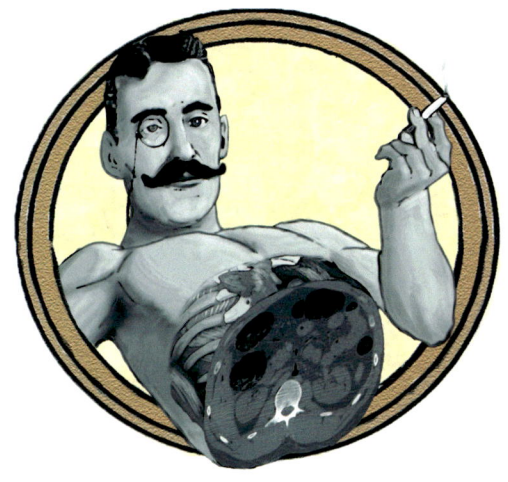

20. **Superior mesenteric artery** (*A. mesenterica superior*)

21. **Inferior mesenteric vein** (*V. mesenterica inferior*)

22. **Splenic artery and vein** (*A. et v. splenica/linealis*)

23. **Psoas major** (*M. psoas major*)

24. **Quadratus lumborum** (*M. quadratus lumborum*)

25. **Erector spinae** (*M. erector spinae*)

26. **Latissimus dorsi** (*M. latissimus dorsi*)

27. **First lumbar vertebra** (*Vertebra lumbale prima*)

28. **Liver** (*Hepar*)

29. **Twelfth rib** (*Costa duodecima*)

30. **Eleventh rib** (*Costa undecima*)

31. **Tenth rib** (*Costa decima*)

32. **Ninth rib** (*Costa nona*)

33. **Eighth rib** (*Costa octava*)

34. **Seventh rib** (*Costa septima*)

35. **Sixth rib** (*Costa sexta*)

36. **Costal cartilage** (*Cartilago costalis*)

37. **Pyloric antrum** (*Antrum pyloricum*)

38. **Jejunum** (*Jejunum*)

1. **Rectus Abdominis** (*M. rectus abdominis*)

2. **External oblique** (*M. obliquus externus abdominis*)

3. **Intercostal muscles** (*Mm. intercostales*)

4. **Transversus abdominis** (*M. transversus abdominis*)

5. **Diaphragm** (*Diaphragma*)

6. **Ascending colon** (*Colon ascendens*)

7. **Transverse colon** (*Colon transversum*)

8. **Left/splenic flexure of the colon** (*Flexura coli sinistra/splenica*)

9. **Descending colon** (*Colon descendens*)

10. **Spleen** (*Splen/lien*)

11. **Kidney** (*Ren/nephros*)

12. **Ureter** (*Ureter*)

13. **Renal vein** (*V. renalis*)

14. **Abdominal aorta** (*Aorta abdominalis*)

15. **Crus of the diaphragm** (*Crus diaphragma*)

16. **Inferior vena cava** (*Vena cava inferior*)

17. **Descending part of the duodenum** (*Duodenum pars descendens*)

18. **Head of the pancreas** (*Caput pancreatis*)

19. **Superior mesenteric vein** (*V. mesenterica superior*)

VIII – The Renal Artery and Vein – L-1/L-2

In this section, the abdomen has been sliced through the intervertebral disc between the first and second lumbar vertebrae, and rotated slightly to the left. Springing from between the folds of the pancreas are the superior mesenteric vessels, and slightly inferior and lateral to these is the inferior mesenteric vein. The head of the pancreas sits medial to the descending portion of the duodenum. Posterior to the pancreas, and anterior to the vertebral column, the renal artery and vein span the midline from kidney to kidney. The small intestines have been removed from the vivisection to better visualize the abdominal contents, however, their position can be appreciated in the corresponding CT.

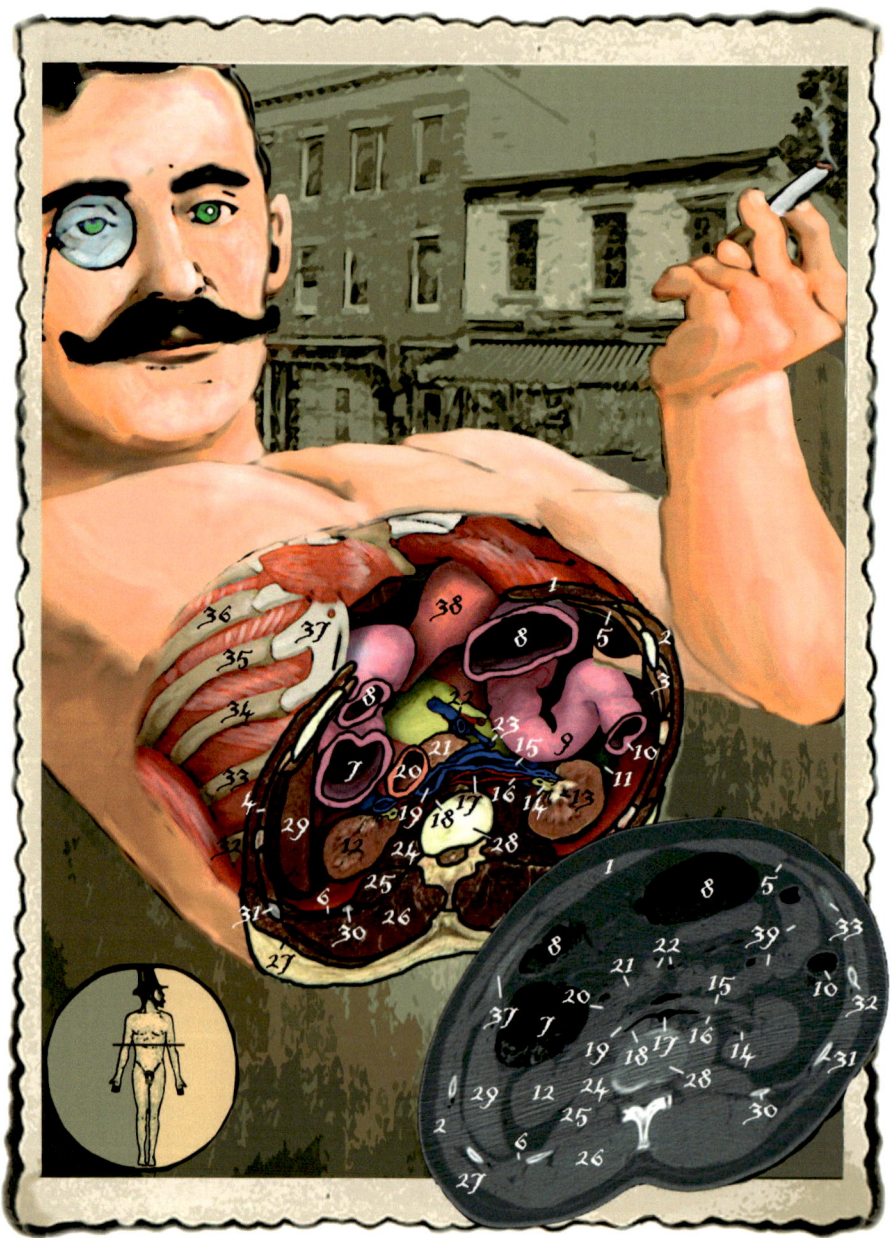

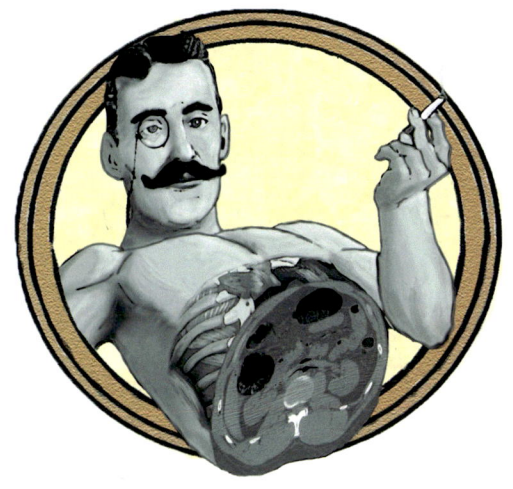

19. **Inferior vena cava** (*Vena cava inferior*)

20. **Descending part of the duodenum** (*Duodenum pars descendens*)

21. **Head of the pancreas** (*Caput pancreatis*)

22. **Superior mesenteric artery and vein** (*A. et v. mesenterica superior*)

23. **Inferior mesenteric vein** (*V. mesenterica inferior*)

24. **Psoas major** (*M. psoas major*)

25. **Quadratus lumborum** (*M. quadratus lumborum*)

26. **Erector spinae** (*M. erector spinae*)

27. **Latissimus dorsi** (*M. latissimus dorsi*)

28. **Intervertebral disk between L-1 and L-2** (*Discus intervertebralis*)

29. **Liver** (*Hepar*)

30. **Twelfth rib** (*Costa duodecima*)

31. **Eleventh rib** (*Costa undecima*)

32. **Tenth rib** (*Costa decima*)

33. **Ninth rib** (*Costa nona*)

34. **Eighth rib** (*Costa octava*)

35. **Seventh rib** (*Costa septima*)

36. **Sixth rib** (*Costa sexta*)

37. **Costal cartilage** (*Cartilago costalis*)

38. **Pyloric antrum** (*Antrum pyloricum*)

39. **Jejunum** (*Jejunum*)

1. **Rectus Abdominis** (*M. rectus abdominis*)

2. **External oblique** (*M. obliquus externus abdominis*)

3. **Internal oblique** (*M. obliquus internus abdominis*)

4. **Intercostal muscles** (*Mm. intercostales*)

5. **Transversus abdominis** (*M. transversus abdominis*)

6. **Diaphragm** (*Diaphragma*)

7. **Ascending colon** (*Colon ascendens*)

8. **Transverse colon** (*Colon transversum*)

9. **Left/splenic flexure of the colon** (*Flexura coli sinistra/splenica*)

10. **Descending colon** (*Colon descendens*)

11. **Spleen** (*Splen/lien*)

12. **Kidney** (*Ren/nephros*)

13. **Renal pelvis** (*Pelvis renalis*)

14. **Ureter** (*Ureter*)

15. **Renal vein** (*V. renalis*)

16. **Renal artery** (*A. renalis*) The renal vessels were named by Sylvius, a 17th century French anatomist.

17. **Abdominal aorta** (*Aorta abdominalis*)

18. **Crus of the diaphragm** (*Crus diaphragma*)

IX – The Transverse Duodenum – L – 2

In this section, the abdomen has been sliced at the level of the second lumbar vertebra and rotated slightly to the left. The transverse colon sits in the midline, beneath rectus abdominis. Posterior to the transverse colon sit the superior mesenteric vessels. The descending duodenum empties into the transverse duodenum around the midline. The inferior mesenteric vein sits just lateral to the lateral aspect of the transverse duodenum. The small intestines have been removed from the vivisection to better visualize the abdominal contents, however, their position can be appreciated in the corresponding CT.

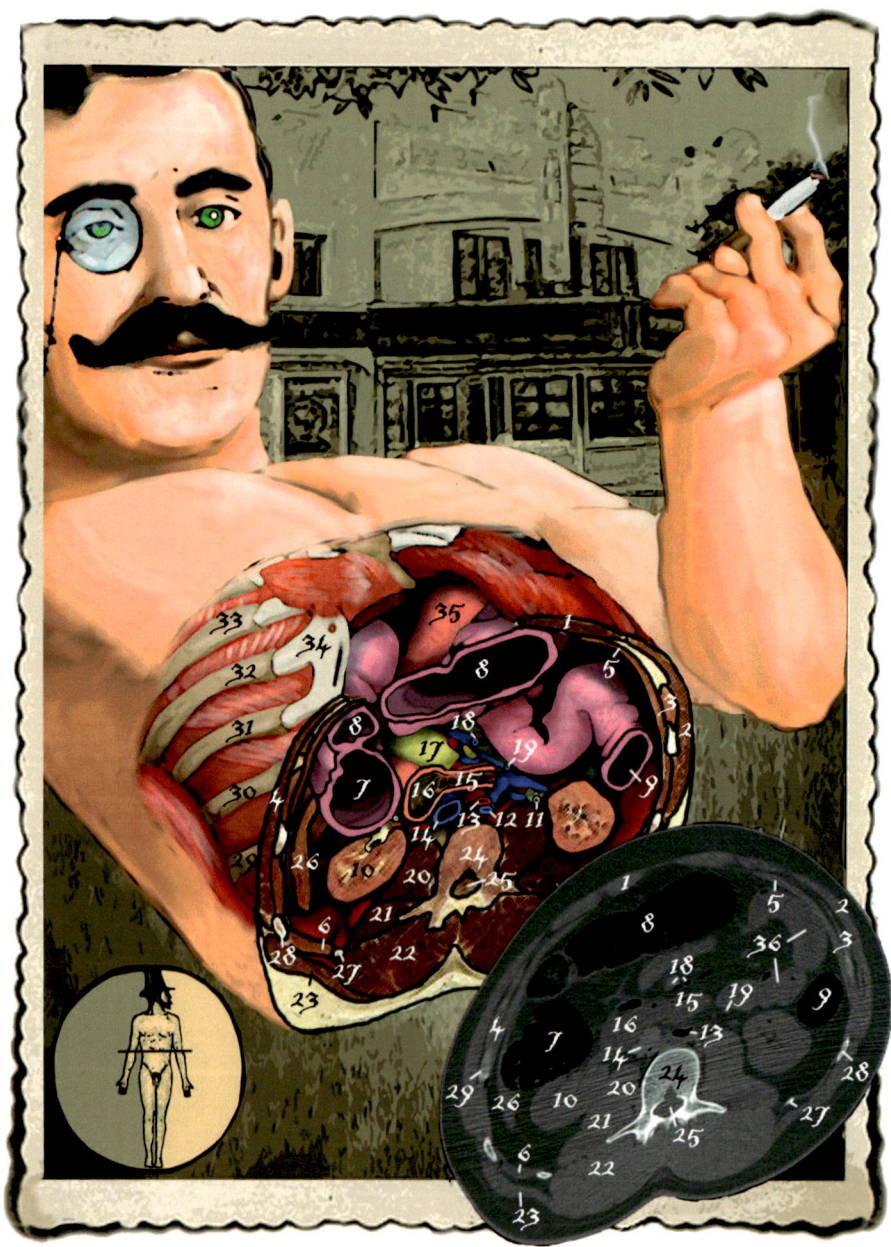

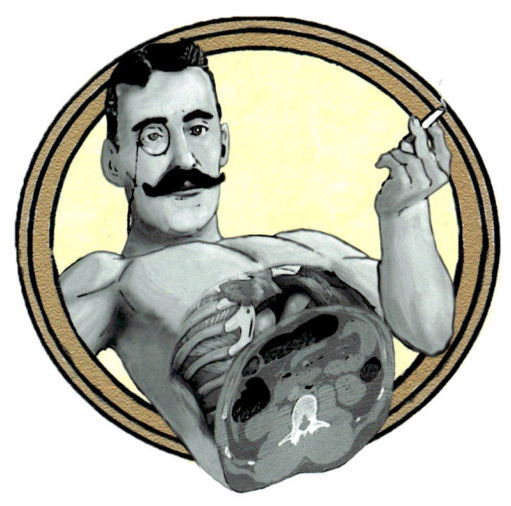

18. **Superior mesenteric artery and vein** (*A. et v. mesenterica superior*)

19. **Inferior mesenteric vein** (*V. mesenterica inferior*)

20. **Psoas major** (*M. psoas major*)

21. **Quadratus lumborum** (*M. quadratus lumborum*)

22. **Erector spinae muscle** (*Musculus erector spinae*)

23. **Latissimus dorsi** (*M. latissimus dorsi*)

24. **Second lumbar vertebra** (*Vertebra lumbale secunda*)

25. **Spinal cord** (*Medulla spinalis*)

26. **Liver** (*Hepar*)

27. **Twelfth rib** (*Costa duodecima*)

28. **Eleventh rib** (*Costa undecima*)

29. **Tenth rib** (*Costa decima*)

30. **Ninth rib** (*Costa nona*)

31. **Eighth rib** (*Costa octava*)

32. **Seventh rib** (*Costa septima*)

33. **Sixth rib** (*Costa sexta*)

34. **Costal cartilage** (*Cartilago costalis*)

35. **Pyloric antrum** (*Antrum pyloricum*)

36. **Jejunum** (*Jejunum*)

1. **Rectus Abdominis** (*M. rectus abdominis*)

2. **External oblique** (*M. obliquus externus abdominis*)

3. **Internal oblique** (*M. obliquus internus abdominis*)

4. **Intercostal muscles** (*Mm. intercostales*)

5. **Transversus abdominis** (*M. transversus abdominis*)

6. **Diaphragm** (*Diaphragma*)

7. **Ascending colon** (*Colon ascendens*)

8. **Transverse colon** (*Colon transversum*)

9. **Descending colon** (*Colon descendens*)

10. **Kidney** (*Ren/nephros*)

11. **Ureter** (*Ureter*)

12. **Tributary of the left renal vein** (*V. renalis*)

13. **Abdominal aorta** (*Aorta abdominalis*)

14. **Inferior vena cava** (*Vena cava inferior*)

15. **Transverse part of the duodenum** (*Duodenum pars transversus*)

16. **Descending part of the duodenum** (*Duodenum pars descendens*)

17. **Head of the pancreas** (*Caput pancreatis*)

X – The Third Lumbar Vertebra

In this section the abdomen has been sliced at the level of the third level vertebra and rotated slightly to the left. The ascending and descending colons sit on either side of the abdominal cavity. The inferior vena cava and the abdominal aorta are anterior to the vertebral body, and the ureters may be seen on either side of these vessels. Note the inferior mesenteric artery as it branches off from the anterior aspect of the aorta. The small intestines have been removed from the vivisection—cut at the level of the distal duodenum—in order to better visualize the abdominal contents. However, their position can be appreciated in the corresponding CT.

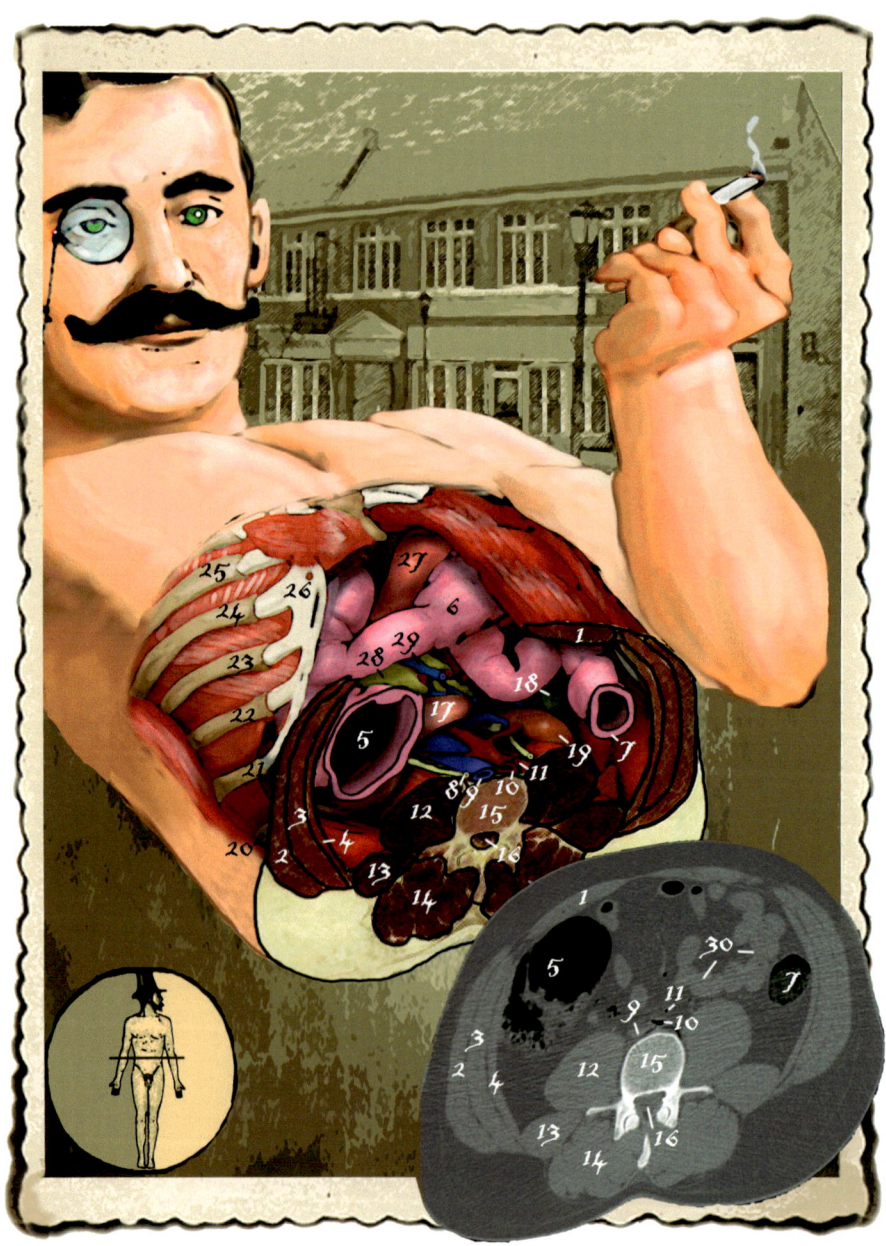

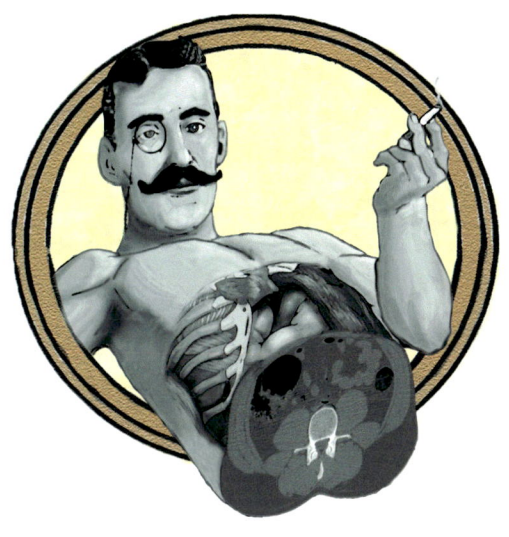

17. **Transverse part of the duodenum** (*Duodenum pars transversus*)

18. **Spleen** (*Splen/lien*)

19. **Kidney** (*Ren/nephros*)

20. **Eleventh rib** (*Costa undecima*)

21. **Tenth rib** (*Costa decima*)

22. **Ninth rib** (*Costa nona*)

23. **Eighth rib** (*Costa octava*)

24. **Seventh rib** (*Costa septima*)

25. **Sixth rib** (*Costa sexta*)

26. **Costal cartilage** (*Cartilago costalis*)

27. **Pyloric antrum** (*Antrum pyloricum*)

28. **Head of the pancreas** (*Caput pancreatis*)

29. **Superior mesenteric artery and vein** (*A. et v. mesenterica superior*)

30. **Ileum** (*Ileum*)

1. **Rectus Abdominis** (*M. rectus abdominis*)

2. **External oblique** (*M. obliquus externus abdominis*)

3. **Internal oblique** (*M. obliquus internus abdominis*)

4. **Transversus abdominis** (*M. transversus abdominis*)

5. **Ascending colon** (*Colon ascendens*)

6. **Transverse colon** (*Colon transversum*)

7. **Descending colon** (*Colon descendens*)

8. **Ureter** (*Ureter*)

9. **Inferior vena cava** (*Vena cava inferior*)

10. **Abdominal aorta** (*Aorta abdominalis*)

11. **Inferior mesenteric artery** (*A. mesenterica inferior*)

12. **Psoas major** (*M. psoas major*)

13. **Quadratus lumborum** (*M. quadratus lumborum*)

14. **Erector spinae** (*M. erector spinae*)

15. **Third lumbar vertebra** (*Vertebra lumbale tertia*)

16. **Cauda equina** (*Cauda equina*)

XI – The Fourth Lumbar Vertebra

In this section, the abdomen has been sliced at the level of the fourth lumbar vertebra and rotated slightly to the left. The external and internal oblique and transversus abdominis are nicely delineated. These three muscles form the lateral aspect of the abdominal wall. Note that in the vivisection these muscles have only been illustrated in cross-section on the left. The ascending colon occupies a prominent position on the left, the descending colon on the right. Anterior to the vertebral body, the inferior vena cava and abdominal aorta are flanked by the ureters. The inferior mesenteric artery branches off from the aorta. The small intestines have been removed from the vivisection to better visualize the abdominal contents, however, their position can be appreciated in the corresponding CT.

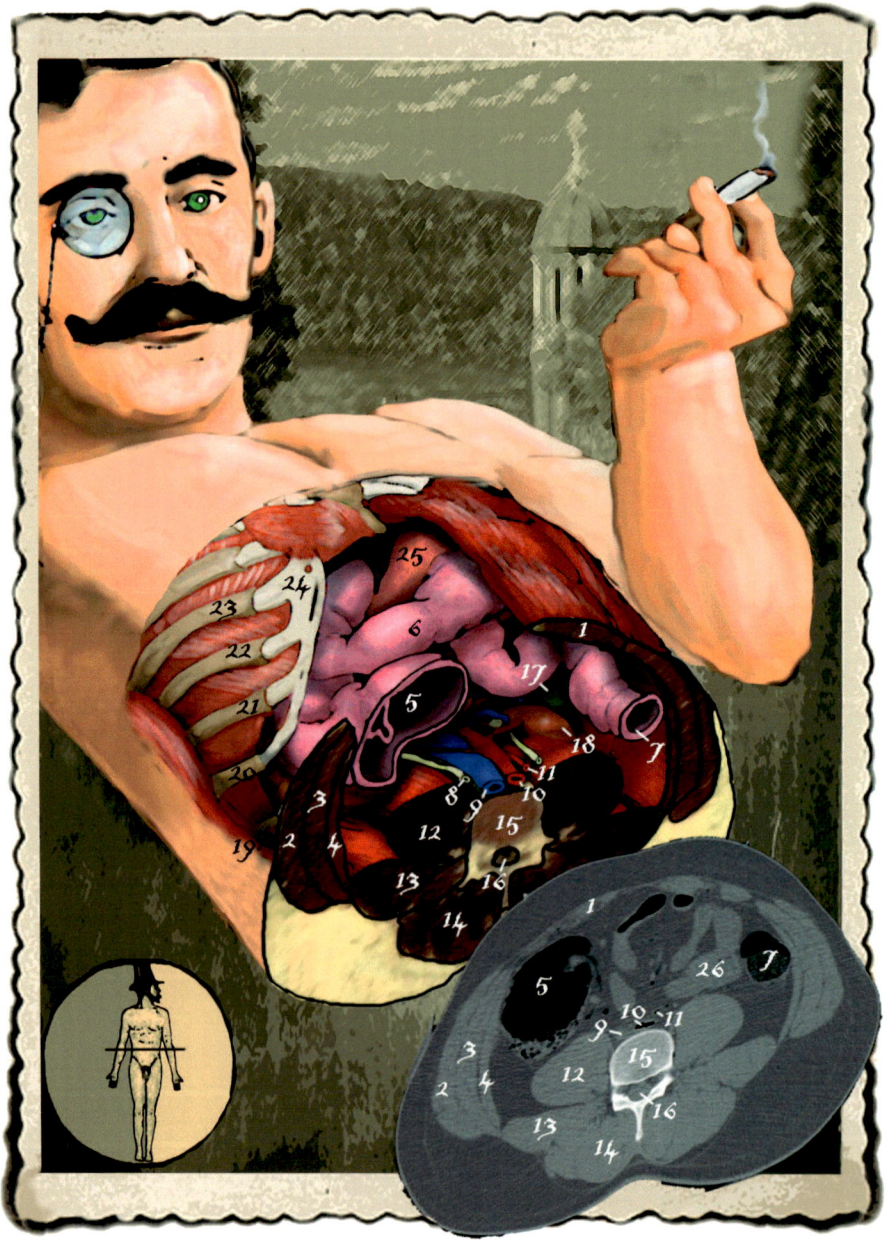

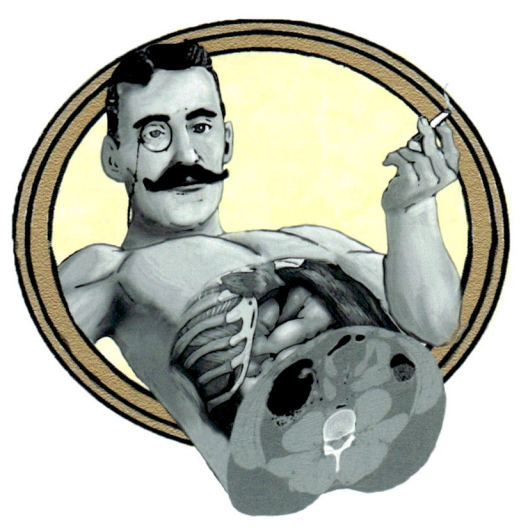

9. **Inferior vena cava** (*Vena cava inferior*)

10. **Abdominal aorta** (*Aorta abdominalis*)

11. **Inferior mesenteric artery** (*A. mesenterica inferior*)

12. **Psoas major** (*M. psoas major*)

13. **Quadratus lumborum** (*M. quadratus lumborum*)

14. **Erector spinae** (*M. erector spinae*)

15. **Fourth lumbar vertebra** (*Vertebra lumbale quarta*)

16. **Cauda equina** (*Cauda equina*)

17. **Spleen** (*Splen/lien*)

18. **Kidney** (*Ren/nephros*)

19. **Eleventh rib** (*Costa undecima*)

20. **Tenth rib** (*Costa decima*)

21. **Ninth rib** (*Costa nona*)

22. **Eighth rib** (*Costa octava*)

23. **Seventh rib** (*Costa septima*)

24. **Costal cartilage** (*Cartilago costalis*)

25. **Pyloric antrum** (*Antrum pyloricum*)

26. **Ileum** (*Ileum*) Derived from, ειλεός, meaning to twist, the twisted gut was so named by Galen.

1. **Rectus Abdominis** (*M. rectus abdominis*)

2. **External oblique** (*M. obliquus externus abdominis*)

3. **Internal oblique** (*M. obliquus internus abdominis*)

4. **Transversus abdominis** (*M. transversus abdominis*)

5. **Ascending colon** (*Colon ascendens*)

6. **Transverse colon** (*Colon transversum*)

7. **Descending colon** (*Colon descendens*)

8. **Ureter** (*Ureter*)

CHAPTER FOUR
THE PELVIS

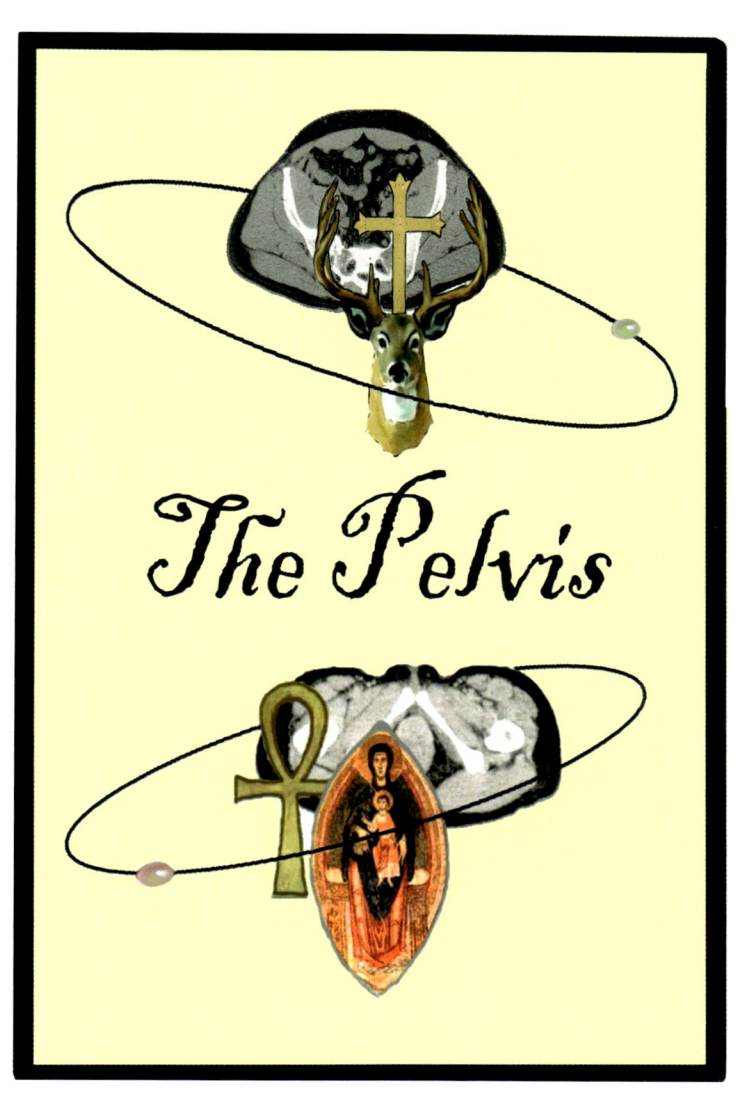

Part One:
The Male Pelvis

I – The Ileo-Caecal Junction and the Sacroiliac Joint – S-1

The pelvis, derived from πύελις, meaning basin, was named by Celsus. Here it has been sliced at the level of about the first sacral vertebra, and rotated to the right. At about 11 o'clock, directly posterior to the rectus abdominis muscles, sits the ileocaecal junction. The caecum is located at about 10 o'clock. The descending colon at about 2, and the ileum portion of the small intestines in between. The cross-section of the sacrum, looking much like a fox face, abuts the ilium at the sacro-iliac joint. The bifurcation of the iliac vessels can also be seen in this section. A corresponding CT shows these structures radiographically.

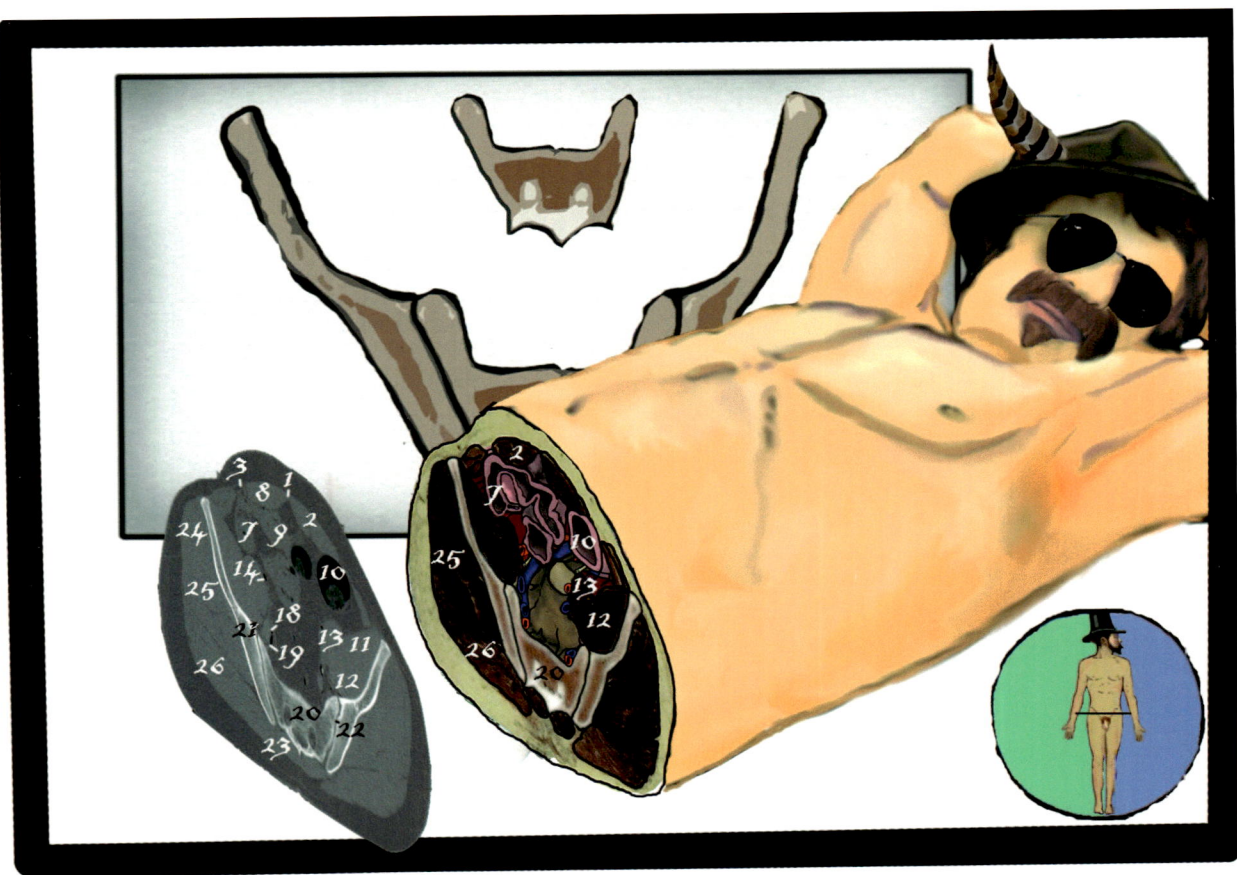

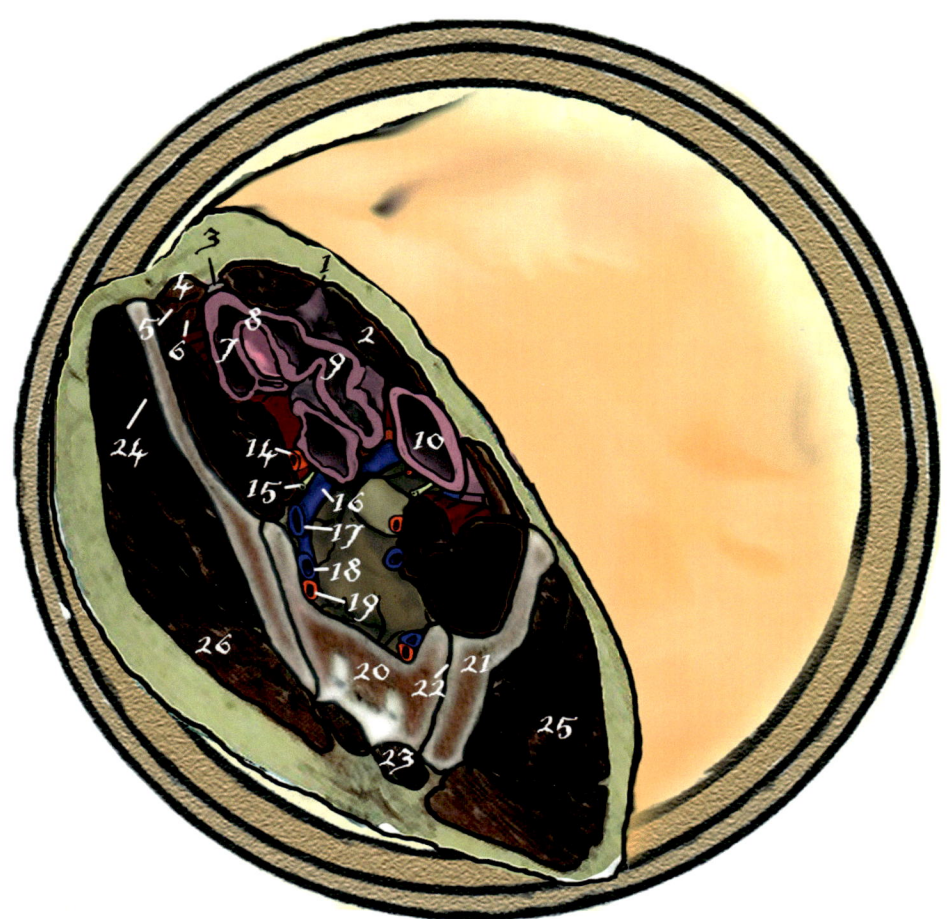

1. **Linea alba** (*Linea alba*) Alba, derived from the Latin term for white, and linea, the term for line.

2. **Rectus abdominis** (*M. rectus abdominis*)

3. **Linea semilunares** (*Linea semilunares*)

4. **External oblique** (*M. obliquus externus abdominis*)

5. **Internal oblique** (*M. obliquus internus abdominis*)

6. **Transversus abdominis** (*M. transversus abdominis*)

7. **Caecum** (*Caecum*)

8. **Ileal orifice** (*Osmium ileale*)

9. **Terminal ileum** (*Ilieum, pars terminalis*)

10. **Descending colon** (*Colon descendens*)

11. **Iliacus** (*M. iliacus*)

12. **Psoas major** (*M. psoas major*)

13. **Iliopsoas** (*M. iliopsoas*)

14. **External iliac artery** (*Arteria iliaca externa*)

15. **Ureter** (*Ureter*)

16. **Right common iliac vein** (*Vena iliaca communis*)

17. **External iliac vein** (*Vena iliaca externa*)

18. **Internal iliac vein** (*Vena iliaca interna*)

19. **Internal iliac artery** (*A. iliaca interna*)

20. **First sacral vertebra** (*Vertebra sacrale prima*) Derived from the Latin, sacer, meaning sacred, the bone was named by Galen. Skinner suggests that the bone was considered sacred as it was believed to be the last bone to decompose and the likely nucleating point of the body during resurrection.

21. **Ilium** (*Os ilium*) A medieval Latin term, Skinner suggests that the bone was so named either because it was twisted, as in ileum meaning to twist, or because the gut can be found resting on it.

22. **Sacro-iliac joint** (*Articulatio sacroiliaca*)

23. **Iliocostalis** (*M. iliocostalis*)

24. **Gluteus medius** (*M. gluteus medius*)

25. **Gluteus minimis** (*M. gluteus minimis*)

26. **Gluteus maximus** (*M. gluteus maximus*)

II – The Femoral Head and Acetabulum

In this section the pelvis has been sliced near the most distal aspect of the coccyx, hemi-sectioned on the left, and rotated to the right. In the midline sits rectus abdominis. Posterior to this is the urinary bladder which is anterior to the seminal vesicles. The round head of the femur sits in the acetabulum like a pearl in a collet. A corresponding CT shows these structures radiographically.

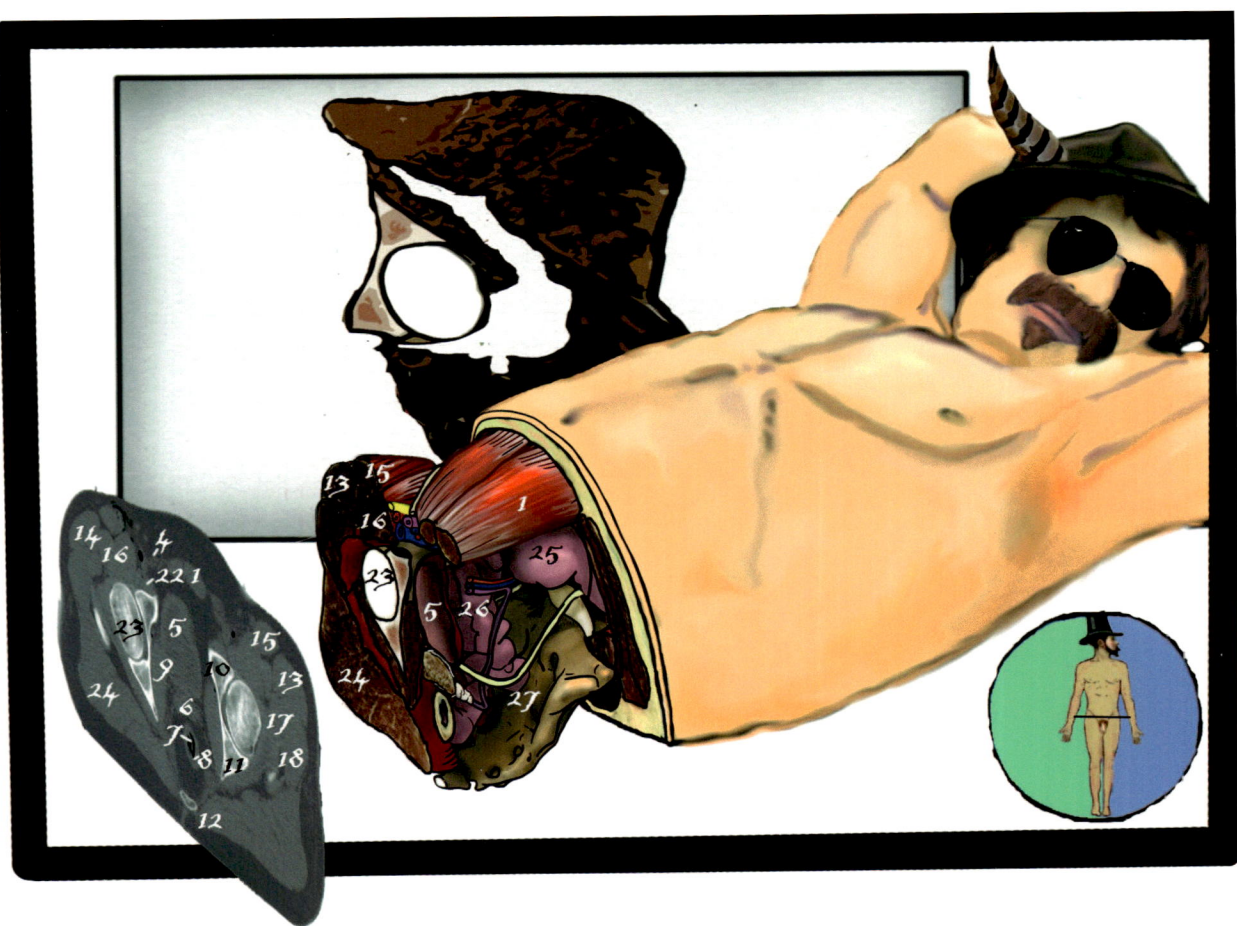

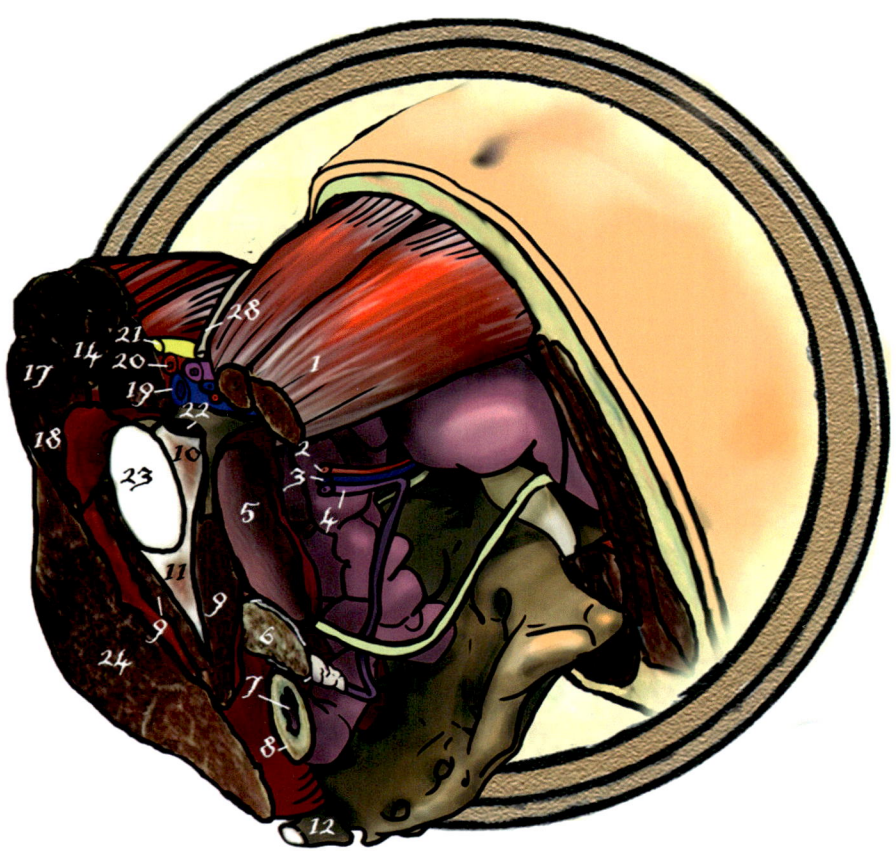

1. **Rectus abdominis** (*M. rectus abdominis*)

2. **Testicular artery** (*A. testicularis*)

3. **Testicular vein** (*V. testicularis*)

4. **Ductus (vas) deferens** (*Ductus deferens*) Derived from the Latin, vas, a term for a container, the structure was so named by Berengarius, a 16th century Italian anatomist.

5. **Urinary bladder** (*Vesica urinaria*)

6. **Seminal vesicle** (*Vesicula seminalis*)

7. **Rectum** (*Rectum*)

8. **External anal sphincter** (*M. sphincter ani externus*) The term anus is derived from the Latin, annus, or a ring, and was first used by Celsus in the 1st century.

9. **Obturator internus** (*M. obturatorius internus*)

10. **Pubis** (*Os pubis*)

11. **Ischium** (*Os ischium*)

12. **Coccyx** (*Os coccygis*) Derived from κόκκυξ, a cuckoo bird, the bone was named by Herophilus in the 3rd century BC.

13. **Tensor fasciae latae** (*M. tensor fascia lata*) Fascia, derived from the Latin fascis, meaning a bundle, or bandage.

14. **Rectus femoris** (*M. rectus femoris*)

15. **Sartorius** (*M. sartorius*)

16. **Iliopsoas** (*M. iliopsoas*)

17. **Gluteus medius** (*M. gluteus medius*)

18. **Gluteus minimis** (*M. gluteus minimis*)

19. **Femoral vein** (*V. femoralis*)

20. **Femoral artery** (*A. femoralis*)

21. **Femoral nerve** (*N. femoralis*)

22. **Pectineus** (*M. pectineus*)

23. **Femoral head** (*Caput femoris*)

24. **Gluteus maximus** (*M. gluteus maximus*)

25. **Descending colon** (*Colon descendens*)

26. **Sigmoid colon** (*Colon sigmoideum*)

27. **Ureter** (*Ureter*) Derived from ουρητηρ, a diminutive on the verb "to make water," the term was first used by Hippocrates.

28. **Linea semilunares** (*Linea semilunares*)

III – The Pubic Symphysis

In this section, the pelvis has been sliced at the level of the pubic symphysis, hemi-sectioned, and rotated slightly to the right. Posterior to the pubic symphysis, in the midline, sit the bladder, prostate, and rectum. The head and neck of the femur may be seen at about 9 o'clock. The acetabulum accommodates the femoral head. A corresponding CT shows these structures radiographically.

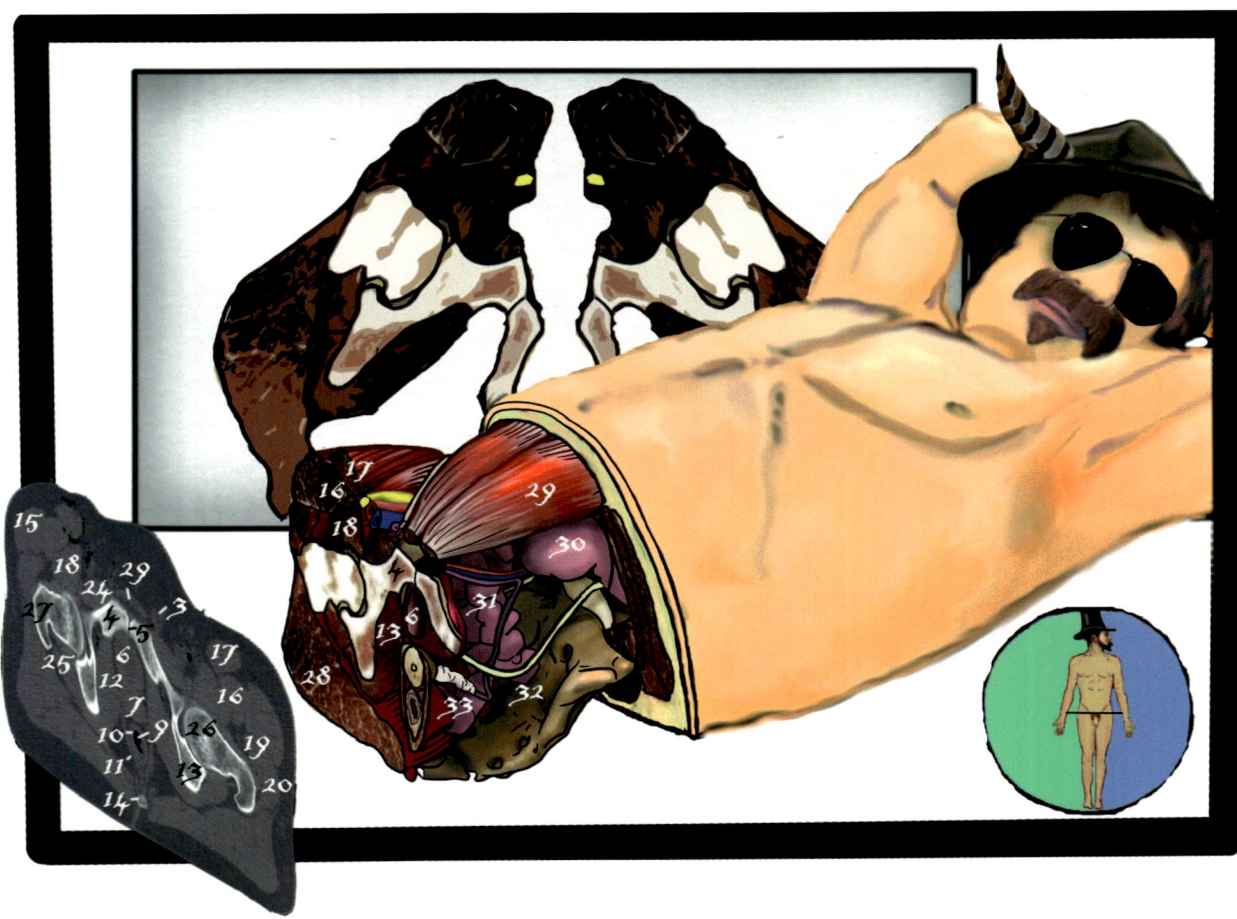

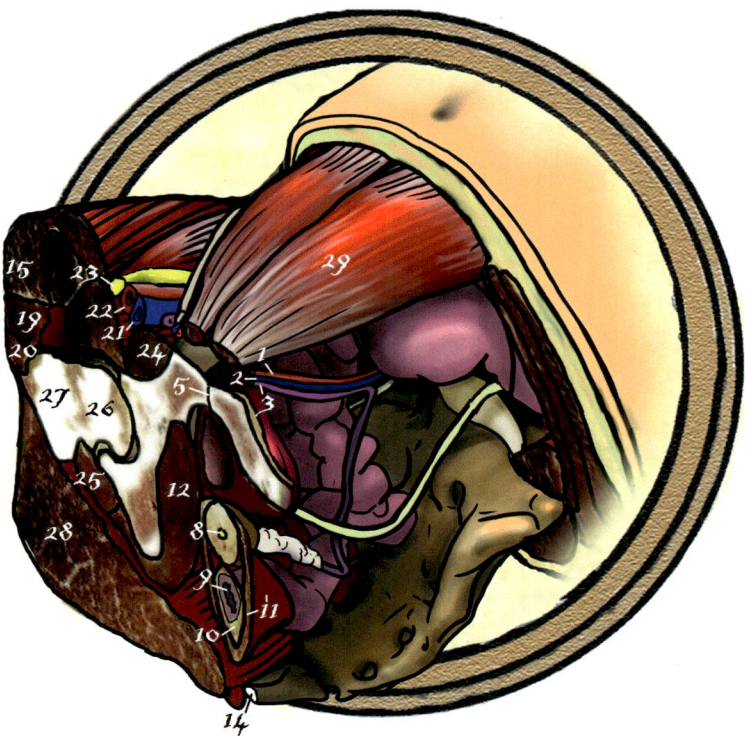

1. **Testicular artery** (*A. testicularis*)

2. **Testicular vein** (*V. testicularis*)

3. **Ductus** (**vas**) **deferens** (*Ductus deferens*)

4. **Superior pubic ramus** (*Ramus superior ossis pubis*)

5. **Pubic symphysis** (*Symphysis pubica*)

6. **Urinary bladder** (*Vesica urinaria*) Derived from blaedre, an Anglo-Saxon term for blister, or a watery swelling.

7. **Prostate** (*Prostata*) Derived from ιστημι and προ, the Greek term meaning "to stand before", the prostate was so named by Herophilus.

8. **Prostatic urethra** (*Urethra, pars prostatica*)

9. **Rectum** (*Rectum*) Derived from the Latin, rectus, meaning straight or upright, Aristotle was the first to describe the straight passage from the bowels to the anus.

10. **External anal sphincter** (*M. sphincter ani externus*)

11. **Levator ani** (*M. levator ani*)

12. **Obturator internus** (*M. obturatorius internus*) Obturator is derived from the Latin obturare, meaning to occlude.

13. **Ischium** (*Os ischium*)

14. **Coccyx** (*Os coccygis*)

15. **Tensor fasciae latae** (*M. tensor fascia lata*)

16. **Rectus femoris** (*M. rectus femoris*)

17. **Sartorius** (*M. sartorius*)

18. **Iliopsoas** (*M. iliopsoas*)

19. **Gluteus medius** (*M. gluteus medius*)

20. **Gluteus minimis** (*M. gluteus minimis*)

21. **Femoral vein** (*V. femoralis*)

22. **Femoral artery** (*A. femoralis*)

23. **Femoral nerve** (*N. femoralis*)

24. **Pectineus** (*M. pectineus*) From the Latin pecten, meaning comb.

25. **Quadratus femoris** (*M. quadratus femoris*)

26. **Femoral neck** (*Collum femoris*)

27. **Greater trochanter** (*Trochanter major*)

28. **Gluteus maximus** (*M. gluteus maximus*)

29. **Rectus abdominis** (*M. rectus abdominis*)

30. **Descending colon** (*Colon descendens*)

31. **Sigmoid colon** (*Colon sigmoideum*)

32. **Ureter** (*Ureter*)

33. **Seminal vesicle** (*Vesicula seminalis*)

34. **Linea semilunares** (*Linea semilunares*)

IV – Mid – Pubic Symphysis and the Prostate

In this section, the pelvis has been sliced at the level of the mid-pubic symphysis, hemi-sectioned, and rotated slightly to the right. The cross-sectioned pubic bone sits in the midline, like a red and white butterfly. The bladder is now superior to the pubis. Traveling posterior, the prostate sits in the midline, the prostatic urethra coursing through. Note the rectum, and how it sits in the sling-like levator ani. A corresponding CT shows these structures radiographically.

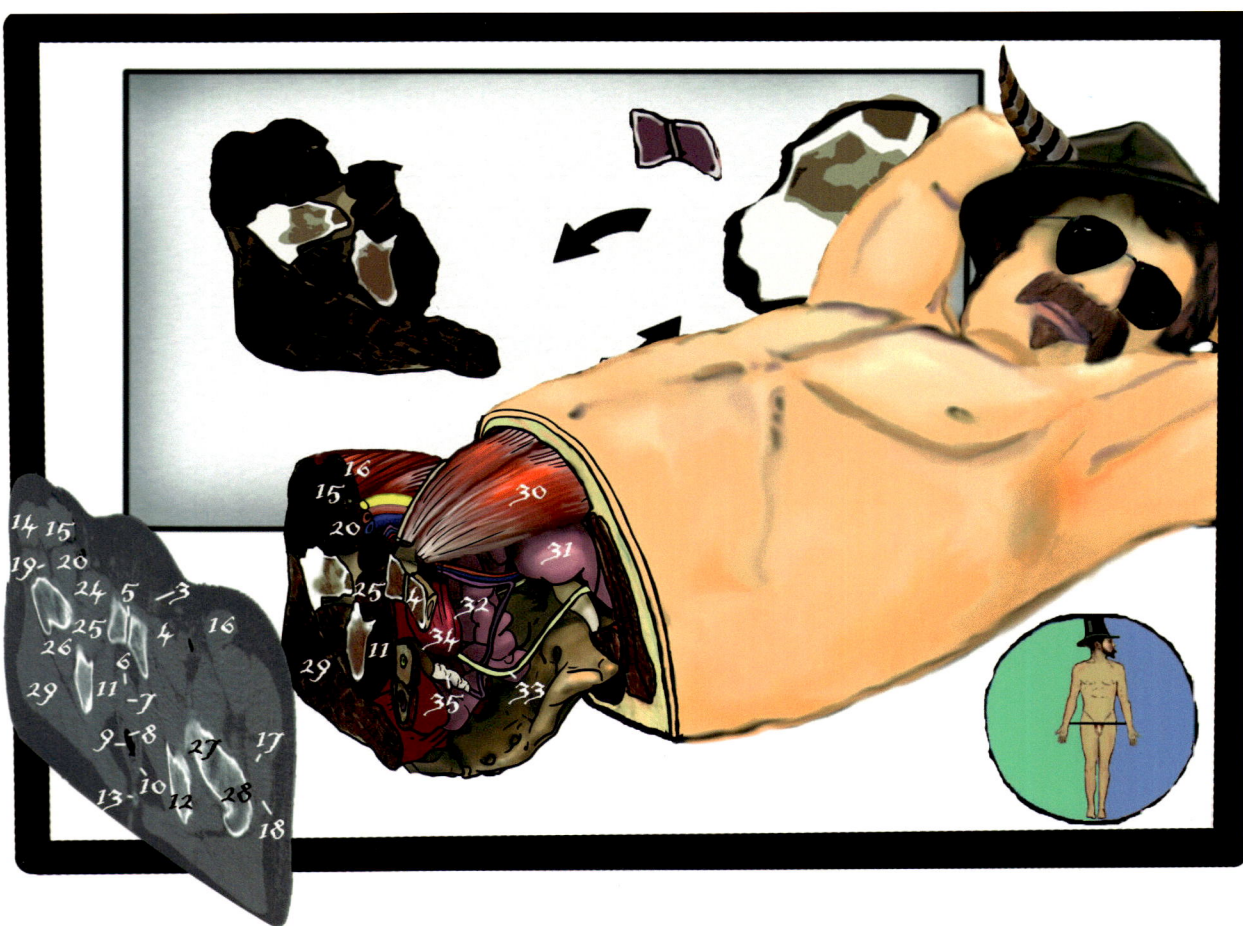

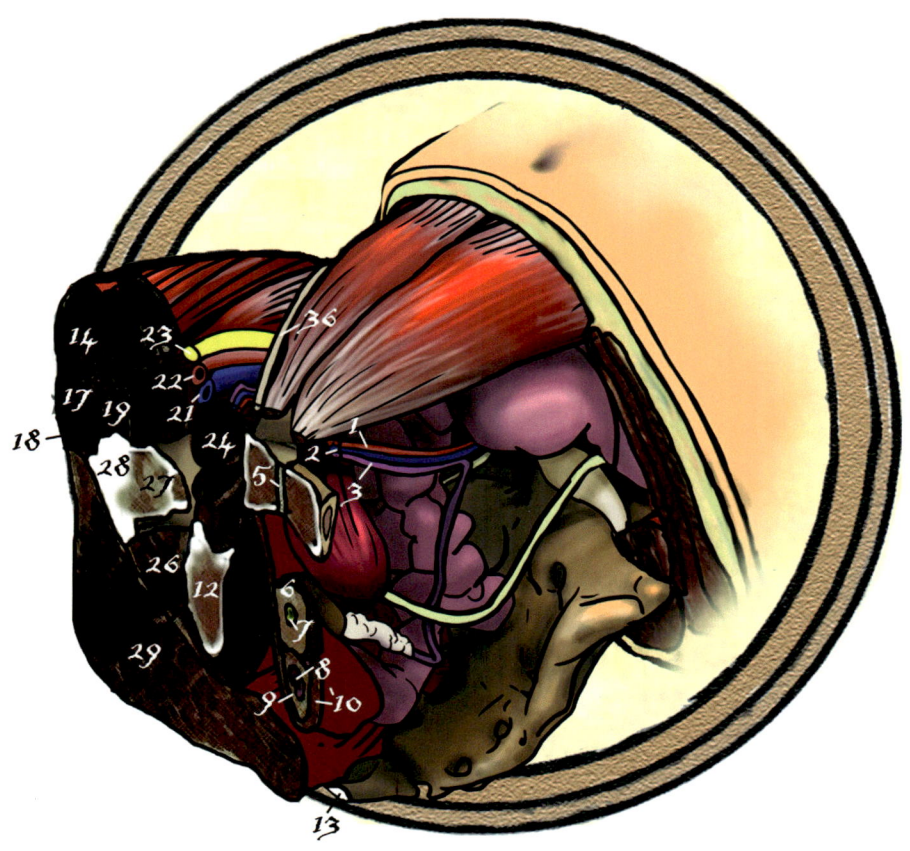

1. **Testicular artery** (*A. testicularis*)	19. **Vastus lateralis** (*M. vastus lateralis*)
2. **Testicular vein** (*V. testicularis*)	20. **Iliopsoas** (*M. iliopsoas*)
3. **Ductus (vas) deferens** (*Ductus deferens*)	21. **Femoral vein** (*V. femoralis*)
4. **Pubis** (Os pubis)	22. **Femoral artery** (*A. femoralis*)
5. **Pubic symphysis** (*Symphysis pubica*)	23. **Femoral nerve** (*N. femoralis*)
6. **Prostate** (*Prostata*)	24. **Pectineus** (*M. pectineus*)
7. **Prostatic urethra** (*Urethra, pars prostatica*)	25. **Obturator externus** (*M. obturatorius externus*)
8. **Rectum** (*Rectum*)	26. **Quadratus femoris** (*M. quadratus femoris*)
9. **External anal sphincter** (*M. sphincter ani externus*)	27. **Femoral neck** (*Collum femoris*)
10. **Levator ani** (*M. levator ani*)	28. **Greater trochanter** (*Trochanter major*)
11. **Obturator internus** (*M. obturatorius internus*)	29. **Gluteus maximus** (*M. gluteus maximus*)
12. **Ischium** (*Os ischium*)	30. **Rectus abdominis** (*M. rectus abdominis*)
13. **Coccyx** (*Os coccygis*)	31. **Descending colon** (*Colon descendens*)
14. **Tensor fasciae latae** (*M. tensor fascia lata*)	32. **Sigmoid colon** (*Colon sigmoideum*)
15. **Rectus femoris** (*M. rectus femoris*)	33. **Ureter** (*Ureter*)
16. **Sartorius** (*M. sartorius*)	34. **Urinary bladder** (*Vesica urinaria*)
17. **Gluteus medius** (*M. gluteus medius*)	35. **Seminal vesicle** (*Vesicula seminalis*)
18. **Gluteus minimis** (*M. gluteus minimis*)	36. **Linea semilunares** (*Linea semilunares*)

V – Inferior Pubic Symphysis and the Ischial Tuberosity

In this section, the pelvis has been sectioned at the level of the inferior pubic ramus, hemi-sectioned, and then rotated slightly to the left. The pubic symphysis sits in the midline. Note the spermatic cord coursing over the left pubic ramus. The membranous urethra may be found in the midline posterior to the pubic symphysis. The left ischial tuberosity is lateral to the rectum. A corresponding CT shows these structures radiographically.

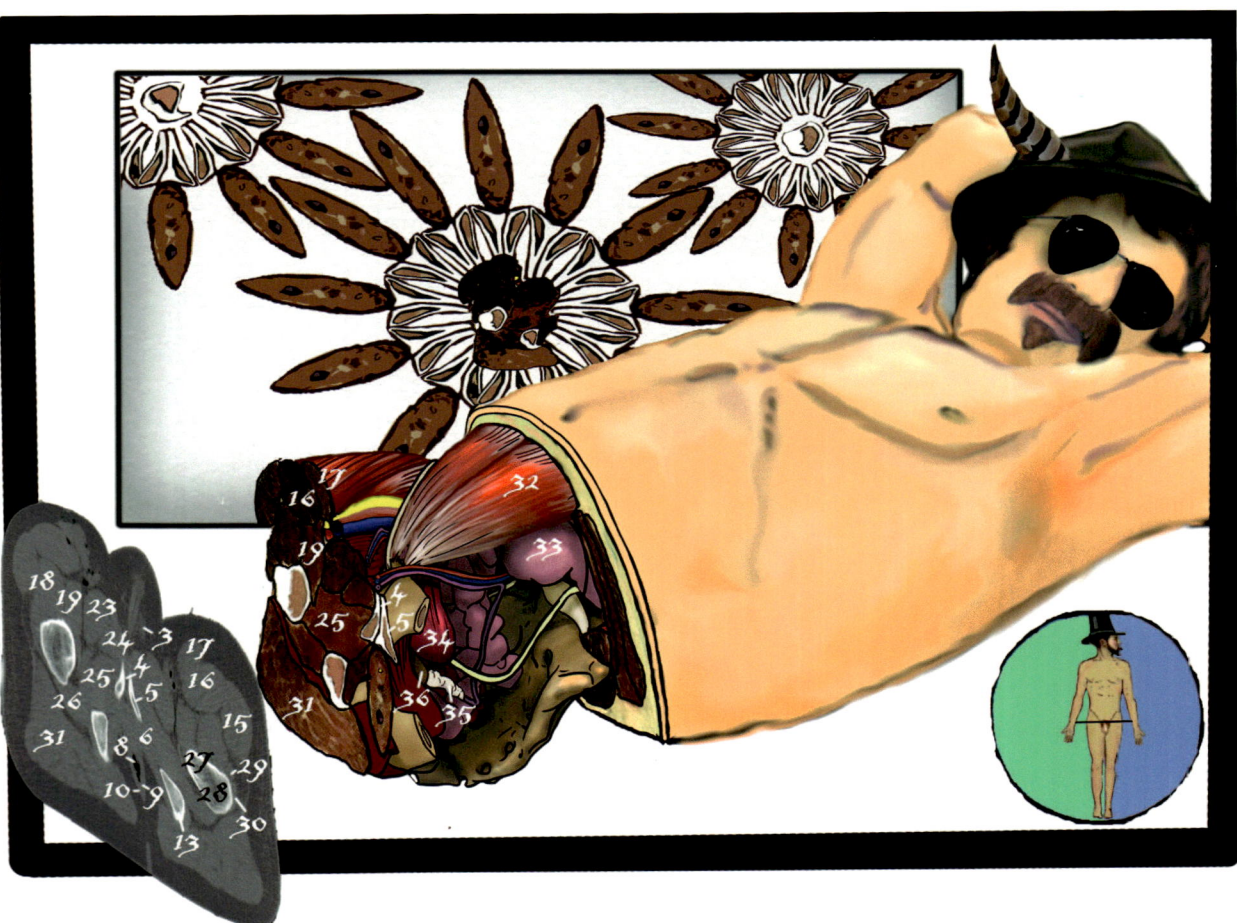

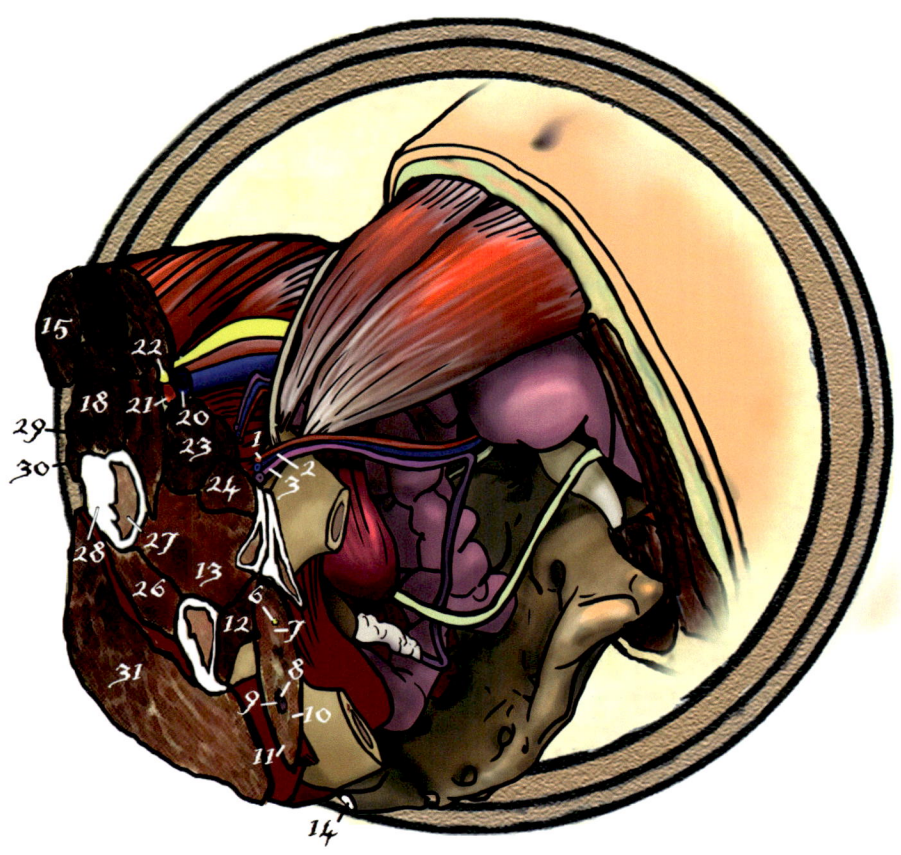

1. **Testicular artery** (*A. testicularis*)	18. **Vastus lateralis** (*M. vastus lateralis*)
2. **Testicular vein** (*V. testicularis*)	19. **Iliopsoas** (*M. iliopsoas*)
3. **Ductus (vas) deferens** (*Ductus deferens*)	20. **Femoral vein** (*V. femoralis*)
4. **Pubic symphysis** (*Symphysis pubica*)	21. **Femoral artery** (*A. femoralis*)
5. **Inferior pubic ramus** (*Ramus inferior ossis pubis*)	22. **Femoral nerve** (*N. femoralis*)
6. **Membranous urethra** (*Urethra, pars membranacea*)	23. **Pectineus** (*M. pectineus*)
7. **Sphincter urethra** (*M. sphincter urethrae*)	24. **Adductor brevis** (*M. adductor brevis*)
8. **Rectum** (*Rectum*)	25. **Obturator externus** (*M. obturatorius externus*)
9. **External anal sphincter** (*M. sphincter ani externus*)	26. **Quadratus femoris** (*M. quadratus femoris*)
10. **Puborectalis** (*M. puborectalis*)	27. **Femoral neck** (*Collum femoris*)
11. **Pubococcygeus** (*M. pubococcygeus*)	28. **Greater trochanter** (*Trochanter major*)
12. **Obterator internus** (*M. obturatorius internus*)	29. **Gluteus medius** (*M. gluteus medius*)
13. **Ischial tuberosity** (*Tuber ischiadicum*)	30. **Gluteus minimis** (*M. gluteus minimis*)
14. **Coccyx** (*Os coccygis*)	31. **Gluteus maximus** (*M. gluteus maximus*)
15. **Tensor fasciae latae** (*M. tensor fascia lata*)	32. **Rectus abdominis** (*M. rectus abdominis*)
16. **Rectus femoris** (*M. rectus femoris*)	33. **Descending colon** (*Colon descendens*)
17. **Sartorius** (*M. sartorius*)	34. **Urinary bladder** (*Vesica urinaria*)
	35. **Seminal vesicle** (*Vesicula seminalis*)
	36. **Prostate** (*Prostata*)

VI – The Ischial Tuberosity and Penile Bulb

In this section, the pelvis has been sectioned at the level of the inferior aspect of the ischial tuberosity, hemi-sectioned, and rotated slightly to the right. Just anterior to the ischial tuberosities, the bulb and crus of the penis occupy the midline. Anteriorly is the corpus cavernosum, the spermatic cord sitting on either side. A corresponding CT shows these structures radiographically.

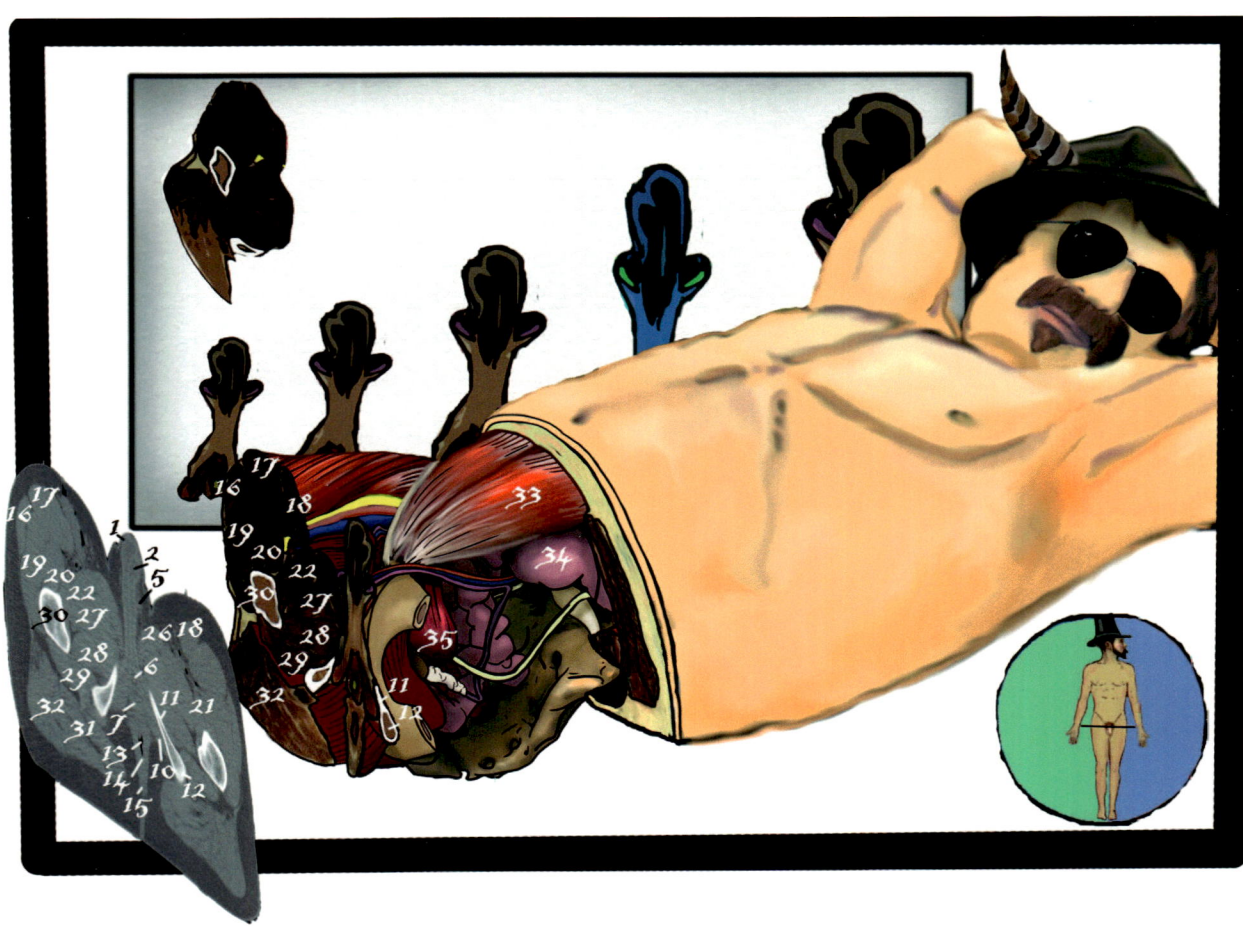

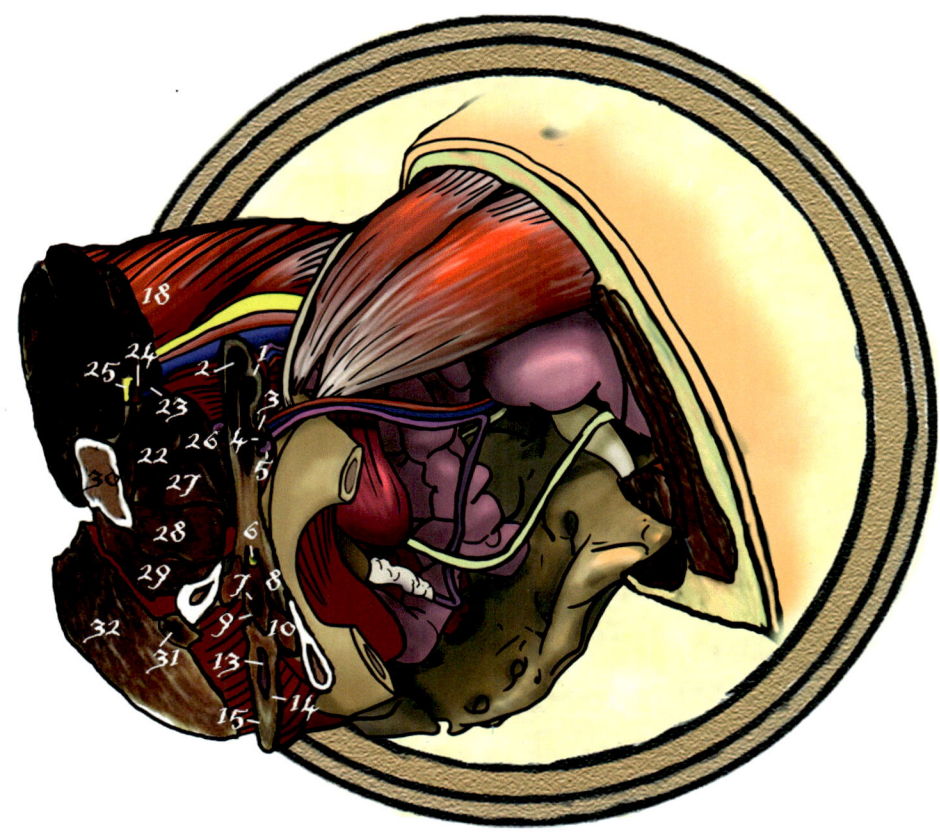

1. **Tunica albuginea** (*Tunica albuginea*)

2. **Corpus cavernosum** (*Corpus cavernosum penis*)

3. **Testicular artery** (*A. testicularis*)

4. **Testicular vein** (*V. testicularis*)

5. **Ductus (vas) deferens** (*Ductus deferens*)

6. **Spongy urethra** (*Urethra, pars spongiosa*)

7. **Bulb of the penis** (*Bulbus penis*)

8. **Crus of the penis** (*Crus penis*)

9. **Ischiocavernosus** (*M. ischiocavernosus*)

10. **Obturator internus** (*M. obturatorius internus*)

11. **Ischium** (*Ischium*)

12. **Ischial tuberosity** (*Tuber ischiadicum*)

13. **Rectum** (*Rectum*)

14. **External anal sphincter** (*M. sphincter ani externus*)

15. **Puborectalis** (*M. puborectalis*)

16. **Tensor fasciae latae** (*M. tensor fascia lata*)

17. **Rectus femoris** (*M. rectus femoris*)

18. **Sartorius** (*M. sartorius*)

19. **Vastus lateralis** (*M. vastus lateralis*)

20. **Vastus intermedius** (*M. vastus intermedius*)

21. **Iliopsoas** (*M. iliopsoas*)

22. **Pectineus** (*M. pectineus*)

23. **Femoral vein** (*V. femoralis*)

24. **Femoral artery** (*A. femoralis*)

25. **Femoral nerve** (*N. femoralis*)

26. **Adductor longus** (*M. adductor longus*)

27. **Adductor brevis** (*M. adductor brevis*)

28. **Obturator externus** (*M. obturatorius externus*)

29. **Quadratus femoris** (*M. quadratus femoris*)

30. **Shaft of the femur** (*Corpus femoris*)

31. **Biceps femoris tendon** (*Ten. m. biceps femoris*)

32. **Gluteus maximus** (*M. gluteus maximus*)

33. **Rectus abdominis** (*M. rectus abdominis*)

34. **Descending colon** (*Colon descendens*)

35. **Urinary bladder** (*Vesica urinaria*)

VII – The Penile Body and Testicles

In this section the pelvis has been sliced in the middle of the penile shaft, hemi-sectioned, and rotated slightly to the right. The body of the penis sits in the midline. In cross-section, the tunica albuginea can be seen enveloping the corpus cavernosum and spongiosum. The spongy urethra sits slightly to the right of midline, near the corpus spongiosum. Superiorly, The penile crus, bulb, and associated musculature sit near the pubic symphysis. The testicles are below the penile body. Although the Visible Man had only one testicle, a second has been reconstructed for illustrative purposes. A corresponding CT shows these structures radiographically.

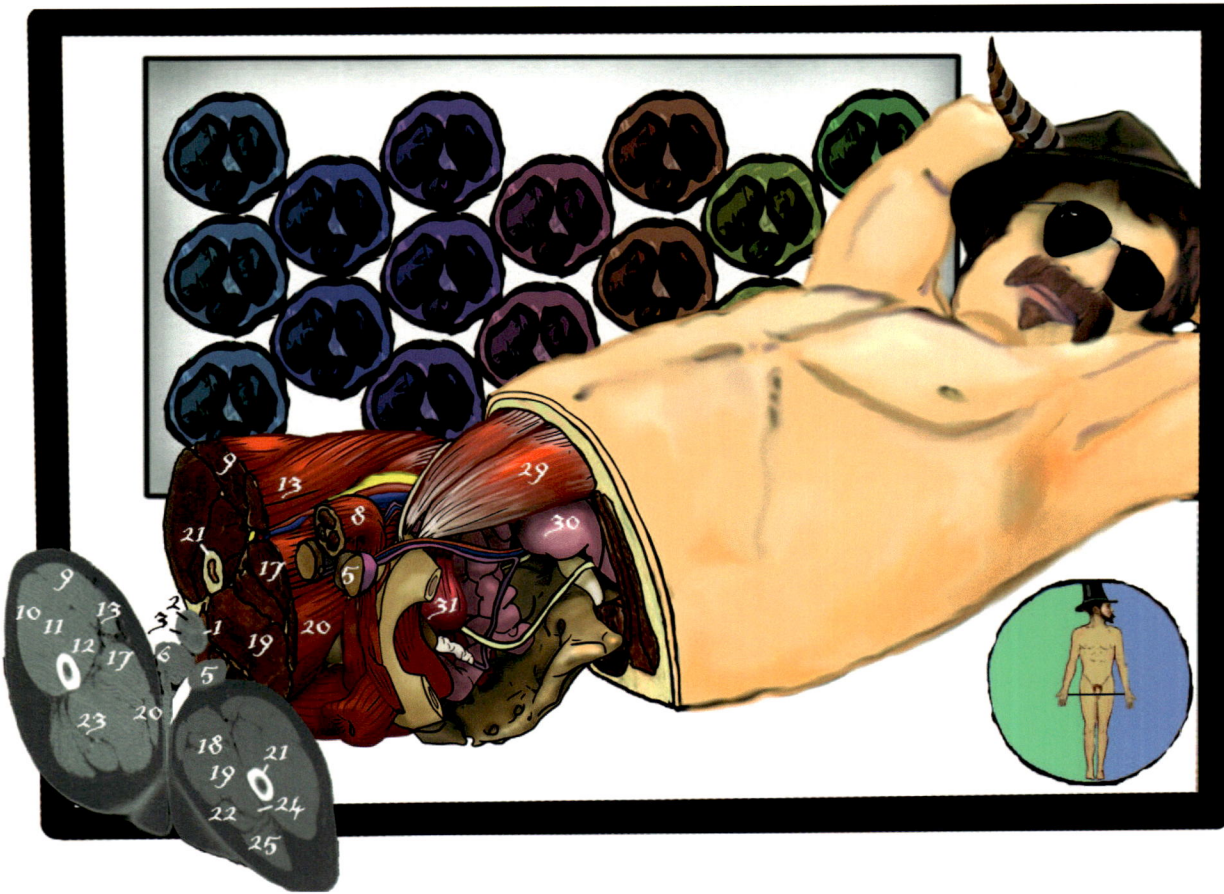

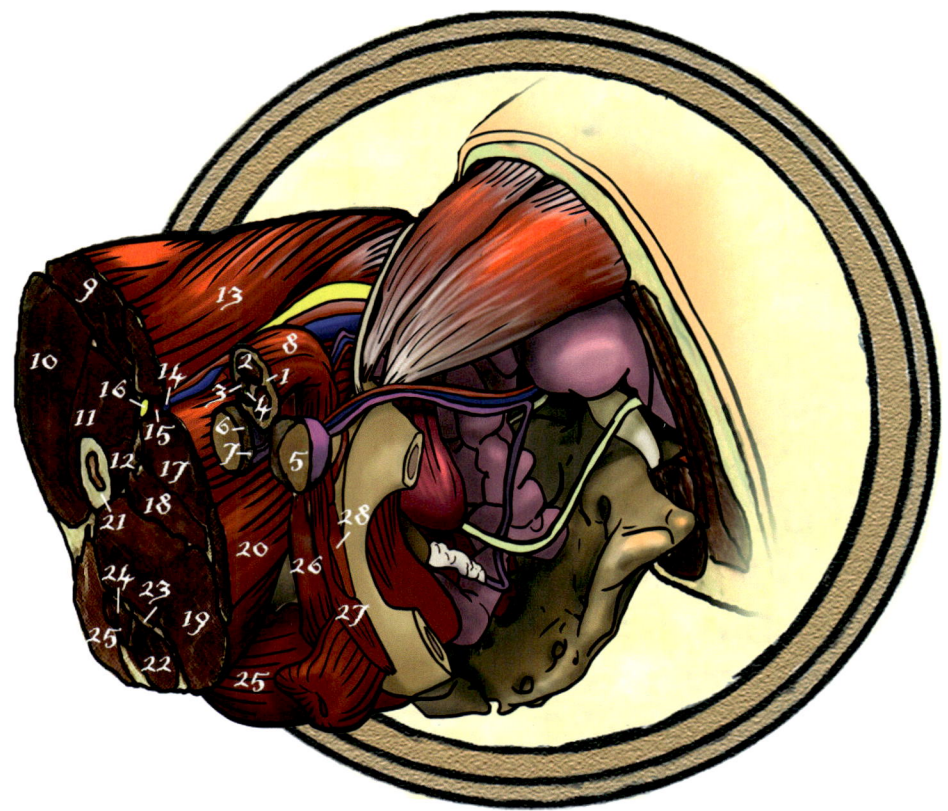

1. **Tunica albuginea** (*Tunica albuginea*)

2. **Corpus cavernosum** (*Corpus cavernosum penis*)

3. **Corpus spongiosum** (*Corpus spongiosum penis*)

4. **Spongy urethra** (*Urethra, pars spongiosa*)

5. **Testis** (*Testis/orchis*) Derived from the Latin, testis. Skinner suggests that the term meant both a testicle and one who testifies in court, and may have been so named due to the fact that under Roman law only men with intact testicles were eligible to testify in court.

6. **Epididymis** (*Epididymis*)

7. **Ductus (vas) deferens** (*Ductus deferens*)

8. **Body of penis** (*Corpus penis*) Derived from the Latin pendere, to dangle down. Also in Latin, a tail.

9. **Rectus femoris** (*M. rectus femoris*)

10. **Vastus lateralis** (*M. vastus lateralis*)

11. **Vastus intermedius** (*M. vastus intermedius*)

12. **Vastus medialis** (*M. vastus medialis*)

13. **Sartorius** (*M. sartorius*)

14. **Femoral vein** (*V. femoralis*)

15. **Femoral artery** (*A. femoralis*)

16. **Femoral nerve** (*N. femoralis*)

17. **Adductor longus** (*M. adductor longus*)

18. **Adductor brevis** (*M. adductor brevis*)

19. **Adductor magnus** (*M. adductor magnus*)

20. **Gracilis** (*M. gracilis*)

21. **Shaft of the femur** (*Corpus femoris*)

22. **Semimembranosus** (*M. semimembranosus*)

23. **Semitendinosus tendon** (*Ten. m. semitendinosus*)

24. **Long head of biceps femoris** (*M. biceps femoris, caput longum*)

25. **Gluteus maximus** (*M. gluteus maximus*)

26. **Bulbospongiosus** (*M. bulbospongiosus*)

27. **Ischiocavernosus** (*M. ischiocavernosus*)

28. **Crus of the penis** (*Crus penis*)

29. **Rectus abdominis** (*M. rectus abdominis*)

30. **Descending colon** (*Colon descendens*)

31. **Urinary bladder** (*Vesica urinaria*)

Part Two:
The Female Pelvis

VIII – The Female Pelvis and the Uterine Fundus

In this section the female pelvis has been sectioned at about the mid-acetabulum, near the sacral-coccygeal joint. It was then hemi-sectioned and rotated slightly to the left. In the midline, the rectus abdominis muscles are tapering off to their distal insertion on the pubic bone. Posterior to these muscles is the fundus of the uterus. The right round ligament may be seen at about 10 o'clock on the uterine fundus, and the uterine tube and ovarian suspensory ligaments sit close by. The ubiquitous broad ligament extends in all directions from the fundus. Posterior to the uterus is the vagina and rectum. A corresponding CT shows these structures radiographically.

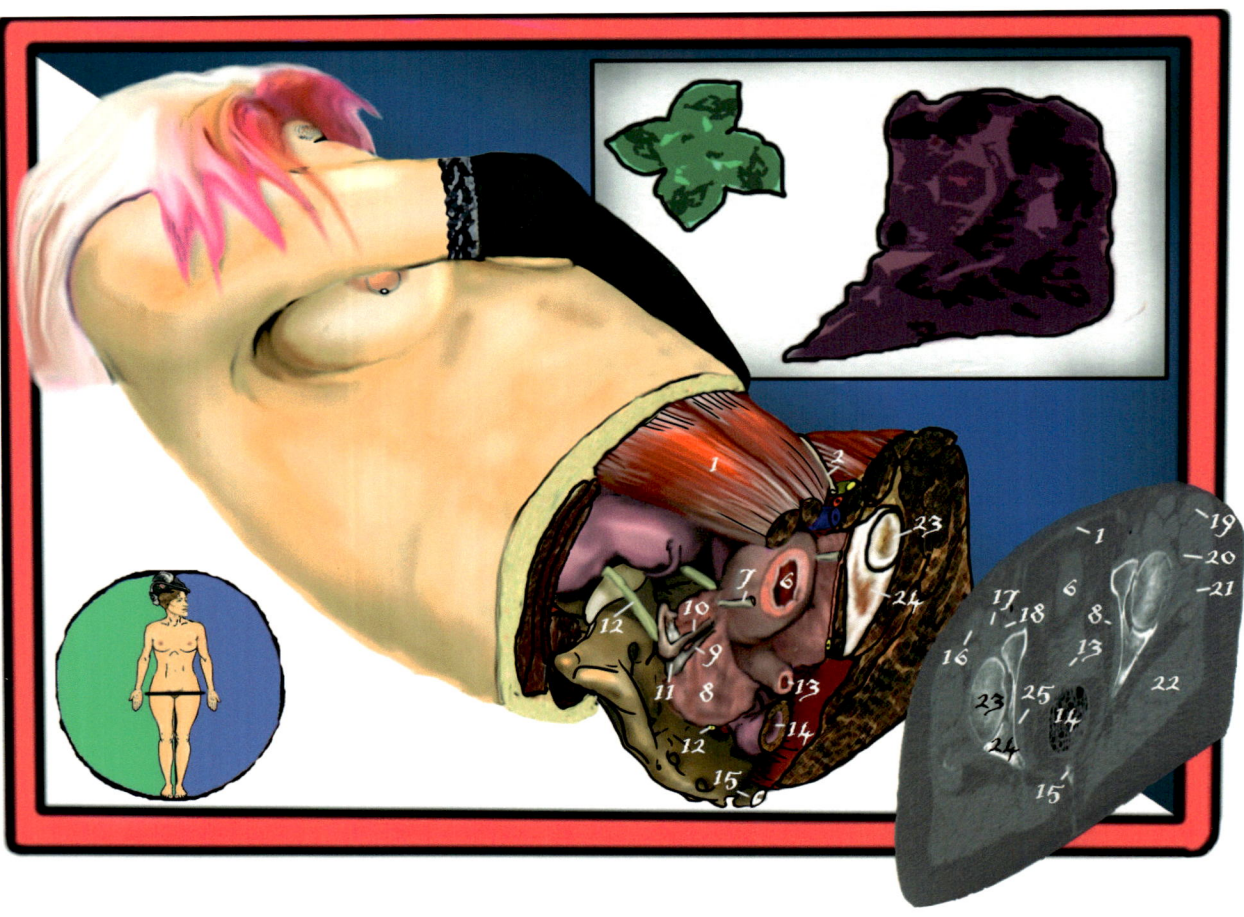

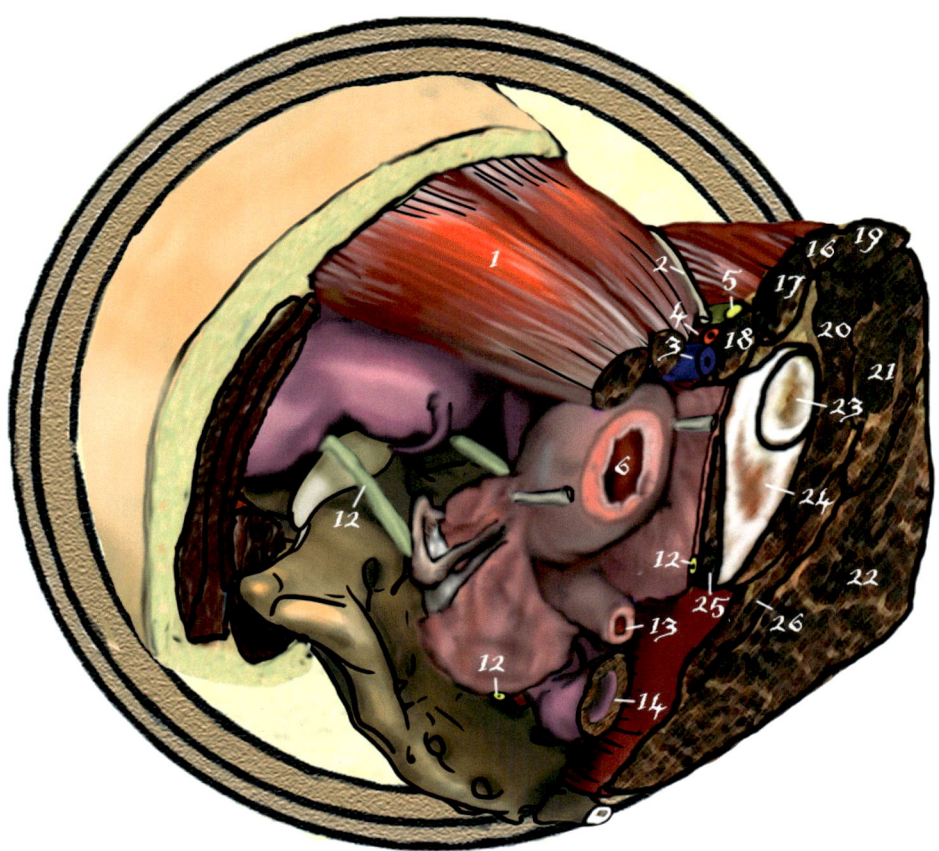

1. **Rectus abdominis** (*M. rectus abdominis*)

2. **Inguinal ligament** (*Lig. inguinale/ arcus inguinalis*)

3. **Femoral vein** (*V. femoralis*)

4. **Femoral artery** (*A. femoralis*)

5. **Femoral nerve** (*N. femoralis*)

6. **Fundus of the uterus** (*Fundus uteri*) Derived from the Latin term for womb. The uterus was also known to the ancients as the matrix and hysteros.

7. **Round ligament of the uterus** (*Lig. teres uteri*)

8. **Broad ligament of the uterus** (*Lig. latum uteri*)

9. **Suspensory ligament of the ovary** (*Lig. suspensorium ovarii*)

10. **Uterine tube** (*Tuba uterina/ Salpinx*) Also known as the Fallopian tube, its eponym, Gabriele Fallopio, was a 16th century Italian anatomist.

11. **Ovary** (*Ovarium*) Derived from the Latin, ovarium, meaning a container for eggs, the ovaries were named by Giammatteo Ferrari da Drado in the 15th century. Many modern anatomy and physiology books describe the ovaries as almond shaped. This is a loaded term when describing any part of the female genitalia, as the almond shaped mandorla was often used in ancient cultures to represent the female reproductive organs.

12. **Ureter** (*Ureter*)

13. **Vagina** (*Vagina*)

14. **Rectum** (*Rectum*)

15. **Coccyx** (*Os coccygis*)

16. **Sartorius** (*M. sartorius*)

17. **Iliacus** (*M. iliacus*)

18. **Psoas** (*M. psoas*)

19. **Tensor fasciae lata** (*M. tensor fascia latae*)

20. **Gluteus minimis** (*M. gluteus minimis*)

21. **Gluteus medius** (*M. gluteus medius*)

22. **Gluteus maximus** (*M. gluteus maximus*)

23. **Head of the femur** (*Caput femoris*)

24. **Ilium** (*Os ilium*)

25. **Obturator internus** (*M. obturatorius internus*)

26. **Piriformis** (*M. piriformis*)

IX – The Female Pelvis and Clitoral Base

In this section, the female pelvis has been sectioned at the level of the base of the clitoris, hemi-sectioned, and rotated slightly to the left. The body of the clitoris sits in the midline, anterior to the urethra. Slightly lateral to the vagina is the clitoral crus. The rectum sits posterior to the vagina. Note the corresponding CT, and compare the more obtuse angle of the pubic ramii.

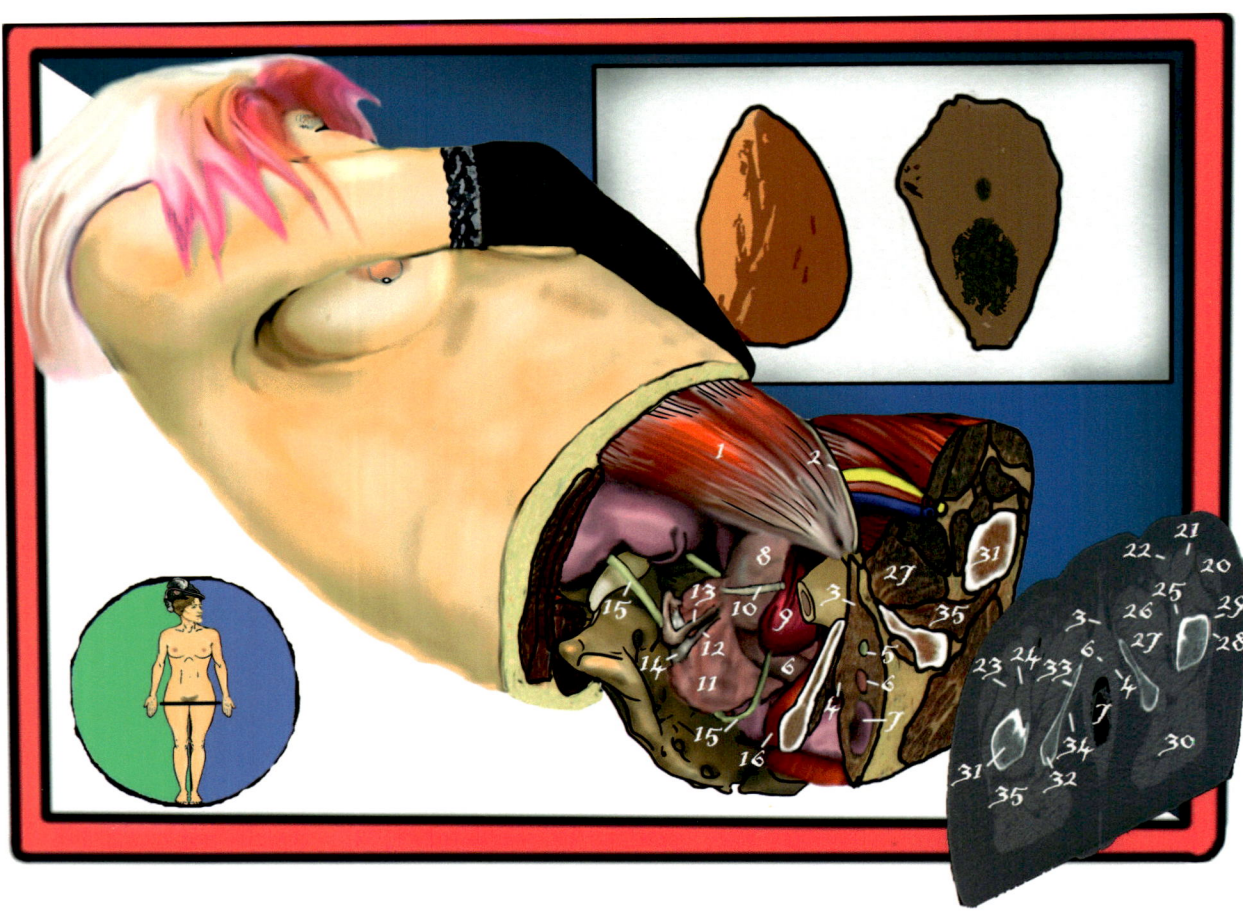

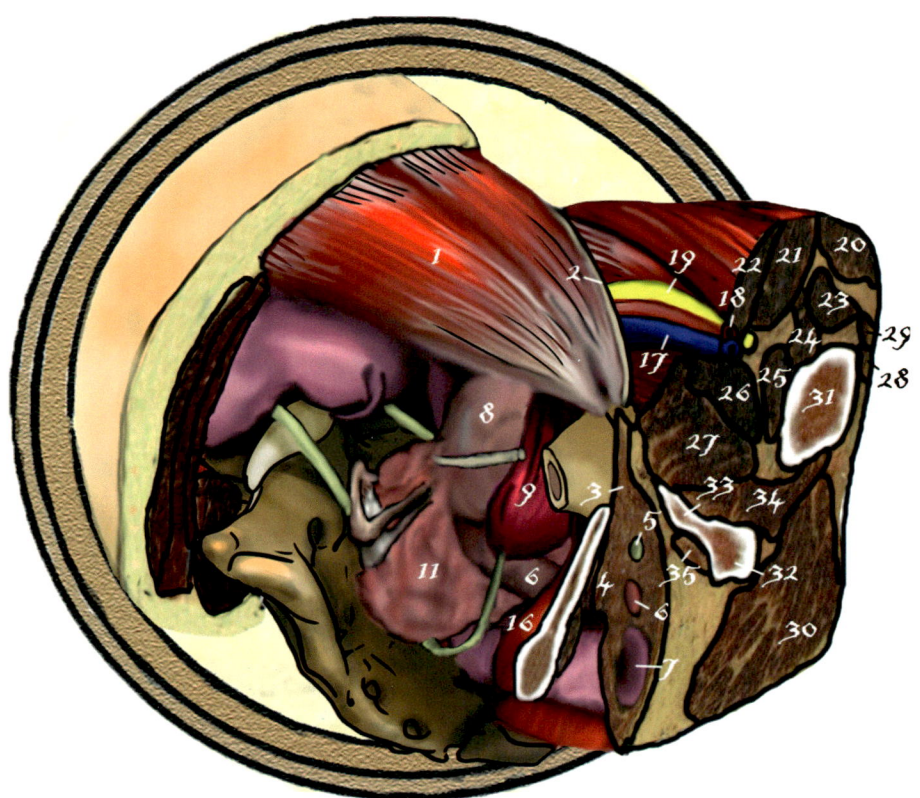

1. **Rectus abdominis** (*M. rectus abdominis*)	**17.** **Femoral vein** (*V. femoralis*)
2. **Inguinal ligament** (*Lig. inguinale/ arcus inguinalis*)	**18.** **Femoral artery** (*A. femoralis*)
3. **Body of the clitoris** (*Corpus clitoridis*) Derived from κλειτορίς, meaning key, or gate-keeper, the clitoris was named by Rufus of Ephesus in the 1st century.	**19.** **Femoral nerve** (*N. femoralis*)
	20. **Tensor fasciae latae** (*M. tensor fasciae latae*)
	21. **Rectus femoris** (*M. rectus femoris*)
4. **Crus of the clitoris** (*Crus clitoridis*)	**22.** **Sartorius** (*M. sartorius*)
5. **Urethra** (*Urethra*)	**23.** **Vastus lateralis** (*M. vastus lateralis*)
6. **Vagina** (*Vagina*) Derived from Latin and meaning a sheath, as in the sheath of a sword. The Latin term for sword, gladius, was a common term for the penis in ancient Rome.	**24.** **Vastus intermedius** (*M. vastus intermedius*)
	25. **Vastus medialis** (*M. vastus medialis*)
	26. **Adductor longus** (*M. adductor longus*)
7. **Rectum** (*Rectum*)	**27.** **Adductor magnus** (*M. adductor magnus*)
8. **Fundus of the uterus** (*Fundus uteri*)	**28.** **Gluteus minimis** (*M. gluteus minimis*)
9. **Urinary bladder** (*Vesica urinaria*)	**29.** **Gluteus medius** (*M. gluteus medius*)
10. **Round ligament of the uterus** (*Lig. teres uteri*)	**30.** **Gluteus maximus** (*M. gluteus maximus*)
11. **Broad ligament of the uterus** (*Lig. latum uteri*)	**31.** **Shaft of the femur** (*Corpus femoris*)
12. **Suspensory ligament of the ovary** (*Lig. suspensorium ovarii*)	**32.** **Ischial tuberosity** (*Tuber ischiadicum*)
13. **Uterine tube** (*Tuba uterina/ Salpinx*)	**33.** **Inferior pubic ramus** (*Ramus inferior ossis pubis*)
14. **Ovary** (*Ovarium*)	**34.** **Obturator internus** (*M. obturatorius internus*)
15. **Ureter** (*Ureter*)	**35.** **Obturator externus** (*M. obturatorius externus*)
16. **Levator ani** (*M. levator ani*)	

CHAPTER FIVE
THE EXTREMITIES

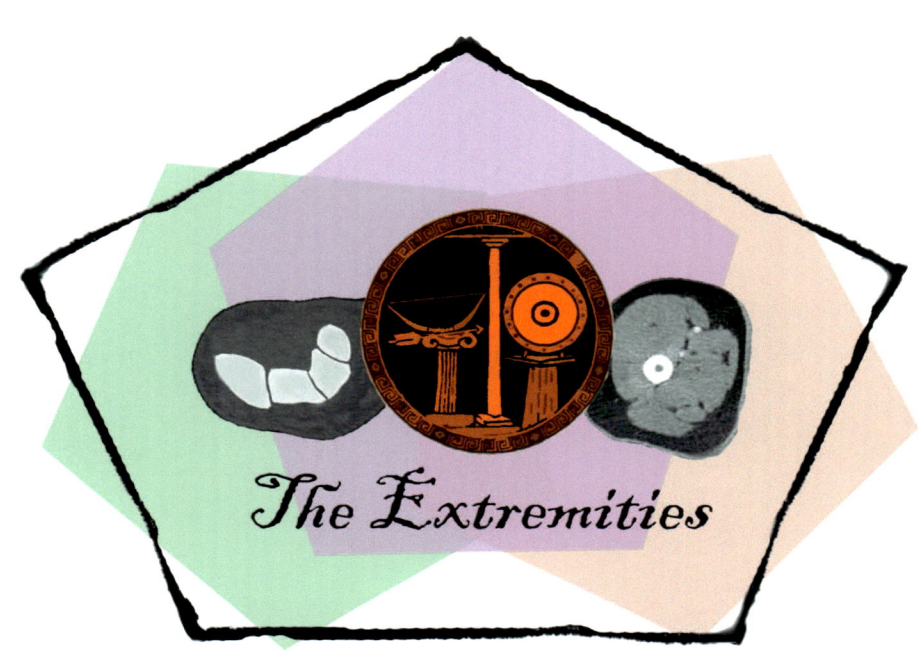

The Extremities

Part One:
The Upper Extremity

I – Mid-Diaphysis- Lateral

The left arm is cut superior to where the deltoid inserts onto the humerus. The inferior aspect of this muscle can be seen as it tapers off into a tendon diving between brachialis and biceps. The cephalic vein can be seen in the 12 o'clock position, and its course traced inferiorly over the anterior surface of biceps. Medially, a wisp of coracobrachialis muscle is seen at 3 o'clock, while, more medial still, sit the more robust of the vessels and nerves that supply the upper extremity. A corresponding MR image has been skewed at the same angle of the anatomic cut. The Visible Human Male was not sectioned in anatomic position. Although it was possible to replanarize the anatomic cuts, the radiological images are slightly oblique. However, this MR does correspond with the anatomic structures, with only slight distortion.

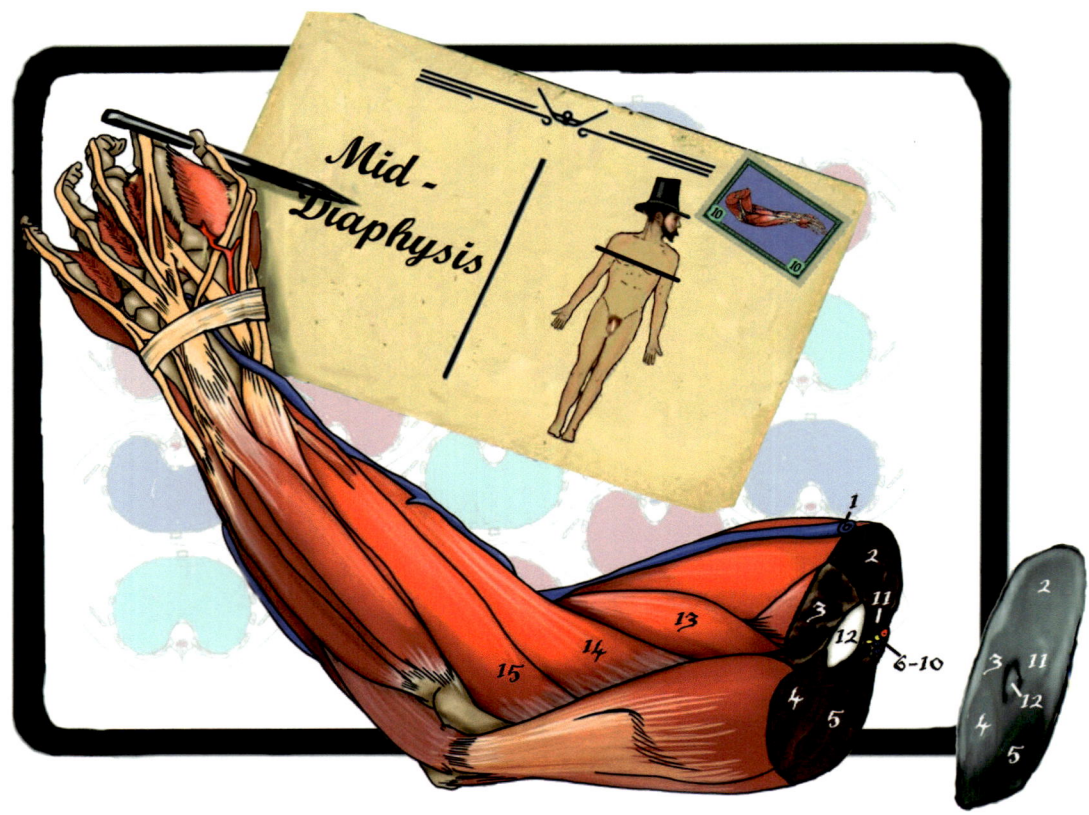

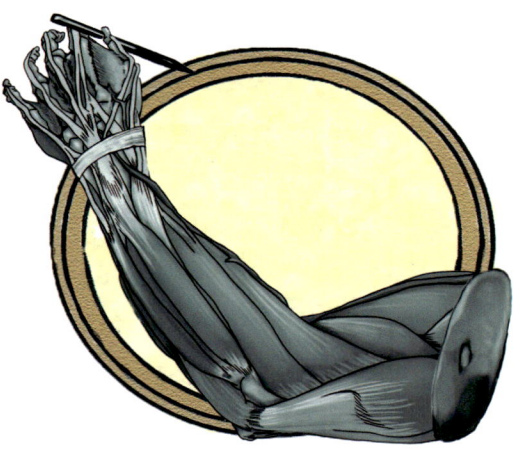

11. **Coracobrachialis** (*Coracobrachialis*) Derived from the Greek κοραξ, a term for something curved like a crow's beak; and brachium, for arm.

12. **Humerus** (*Humerus*)

13. **Brachialis** (*M. brachialis*)

14. **Brachioradialis** (*M. brachioradialis*)

15. **Extensor carpi radialis longus et brevis** (*M. extensor carpi radialis longus et brevis*)

1. **Cephalic vein** (*V. cephalica*) A transliteration of the Arabic, al-kifal, meaning outer-vein. It is a homonym, not a derivative, of the Greek, κεφαλη, meaning head, as the vein was known to the Greeks as the vein of the arm.

2. **Biceps brachii** (*M. biceps brachii*) Named by Albinus in the 18th century, the term is derived from the Latin terms for two (bis) and head (caput).

3. **Deltoid** (*M. deltoideus*) Named by Riolan in the 17th century for the fourth letter of the Greek alphabet, Δ.

4. **Lateral head of the triceps** (*M. triceps brachii, caput laterale*)

5. **Medial/deep and Long heads of the triceps** (*M. triceps brachii, caput mediale/profundum*)

6. **Median nerve** (*N. medianus*)

7. **Basilic vein** (*V. basilica*) A transliteration of the Arabic al-basilik, meaning inner vein. It was known to the Greeks as both the vena internal and the hepatic vein, as it was the vessel opened in blood lettings to cure liver disease. The term is a homonym, though not a derivative, of the Greek word for king, basilica.

8. **Brachial veins** (*V. brachialis*)

9. **Ulnar nerve** (*N. ulnaris*)

10. **Brachial artery** (*Arteria brachialis*)

II – Mid-Diaphysis – Medial

This cut shows the medial aspect of the arm, and is just slightly inferior to the section in I – A. The vessels and nerves that supply the upper extremity can be seen medially, at about 3 o'clock. The brachial artery and vein course into the cubital fossa; the median nerve is seen on its way to dive deep below the muscles in the forearm, while the ulnar nerve wraps around the elbow, just before it hides in the cubital tunnel. Posteriorly, all three heads of triceps are distinguishable, as is a sliver of brachialis laterally. The MR image corresponds with the anatomic structures.

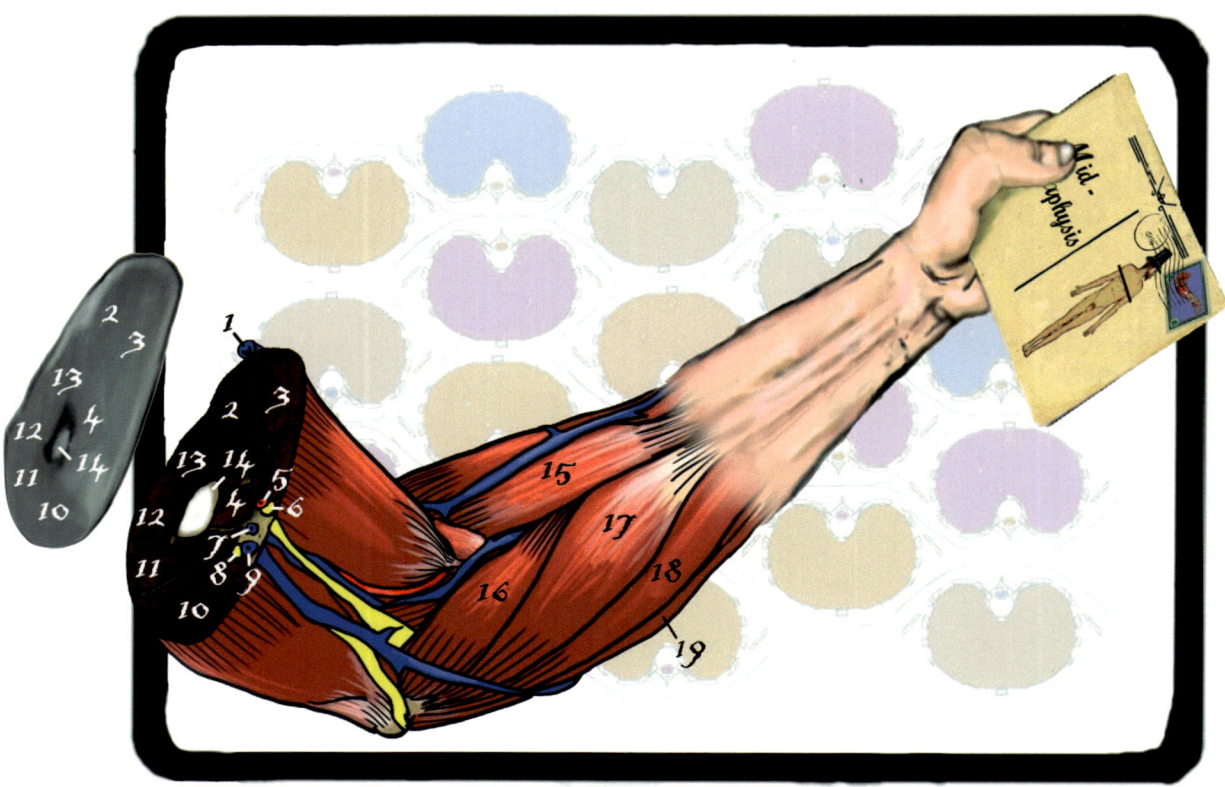

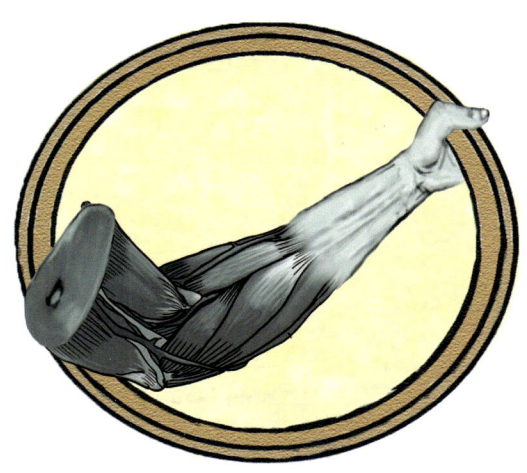

forward, the muscle was named by Soemmering, a prolific anatomist of the late 18th and early 19th century.

17. **Flexor carpi radialis and palmaris longus** (*M. flexor carpi radialis et palmaris longus*)

18. **Flexor digitorum superficialis** (*M. flexor digitorum superficialis*)

19. **Flexor carpi ulnaris** (*M. flexor carpi ulnaris*)

1. **Cephalic vein** (*V. cephalica*)

2. **Biceps brachii, long head** (*M. biceps brachii, caput longum*)

3. **Biceps brachii, short head** (*M. biceps brachii caput breve*)

4. **Coracobrachialis** (*Coracobrachialis*)

5. **Brachial artery** (*Arteria brachialis*)

6. **Median nerve** (*N. medianus*)

7. **Brachial vein** (*V. brachialis*)

8. **Ulnar nerve** (*N. ulnaris*)

9. **Basilic vein** (*V. basilica*)

10. **Long head of the triceps** (*M. triceps brachii, caput longum*

11. **Medial/deep head of the triceps** (*M. triceps brachii, caput mediale/profundum*)

12. **Lateral head of the triceps** (*M. triceps brachii, caput laterale*)

13. **Brachialis** (*M. brachialis*)

14. **Humerus** (*Humerus*) Latin term for the arm bone first used by Celsus in the 1st century.

15. **Brachioradialis** (*M. brachioradialis*)

16. **Pronator teres** (*M. pronator teres*) Derived from the Latin term pronatus, meaning turned

III – Distal Humeral Shaft – Lateral

This section is just superior to the cubital fossa and the elbow joint. Biceps brachii is seen posterior to the cephalic vein. The vessels and nerves supplying the upper extremity are seen medially, while all three heads of triceps sit posteriorly. The lateral epicondyle of the humerus is visible just anterior to the triceps tendon, as is the olecranon process of the ulna. The radiograph is the corresponding MR.

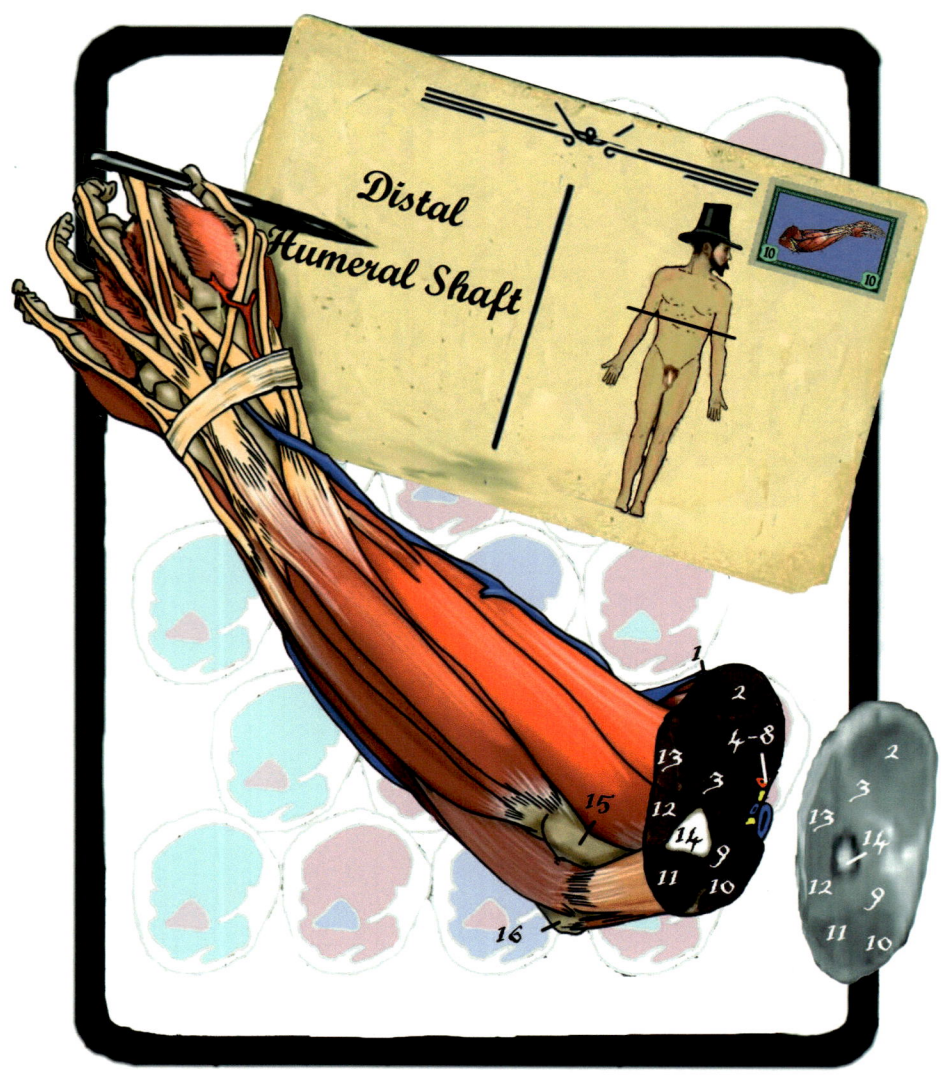

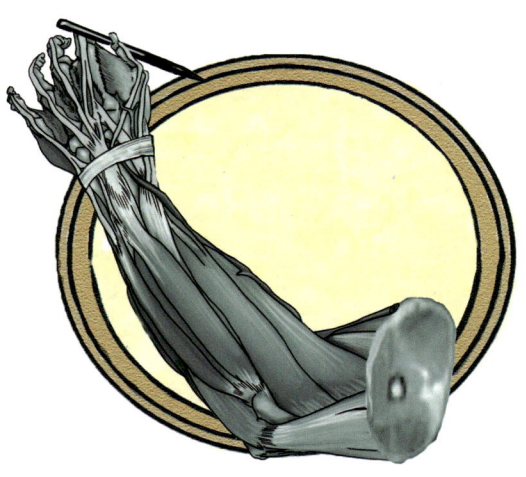

12. **Extensor carpi radialis longus et brevis** (*M. extensor carpi radialis longus et brevis*)

13. **Brachioradialis** (*M. brachioradialis*)

14. **Humerus** (*Humerus*)

15. **Lateral epicondyle of the humerus** (*Epicondylus lateralis*)

16. **Olecranon** (*Olecranon*)

1. **Cephalic vein** (*V. cephalica*)

2. **Biceps brachii** (*M. biceps brachii, caput breve*)

3. **Brachialis** (*M. brachialis*)

4. **Brachial artery** (*Arteria brachialis*)

5. **Median nerve** (*N. medianus*)

6. **Brachial vein** (*V. brachialis*)

7. **Ulnar nerve** (*N. ulnaris*)

8. **Basilic vein** (*V. basilica*)

9. **Medial/deep head of the triceps** (*M. triceps brachii, caput mediale/profundus*)

10. **Long head of the triceps** (*M. triceps brachii, caput longus*)

11. **Lateral head of the triceps** (*M. triceps brachii, caput laterale*)

IV – Distal Humeral Shaft-Medial

This section is slightly inferior to III, and shows the medial aspect of structures seen in a cross-section of the inferior arm. The cephalic vein, still at 12 o'clock, is seen anterior to biceps. Medially, the brachial artery and vein are seen just before they head into the cubital fossa to diverge into the radial and ulnar vessels. The basilic vein courses around the elbow medial to the median nerve, while the ulnar nerve dives behind the medial epicondyle on its way to more distal innervations. Triceps inserts on the olecranon. An MR corresponds to the anatomic structures.

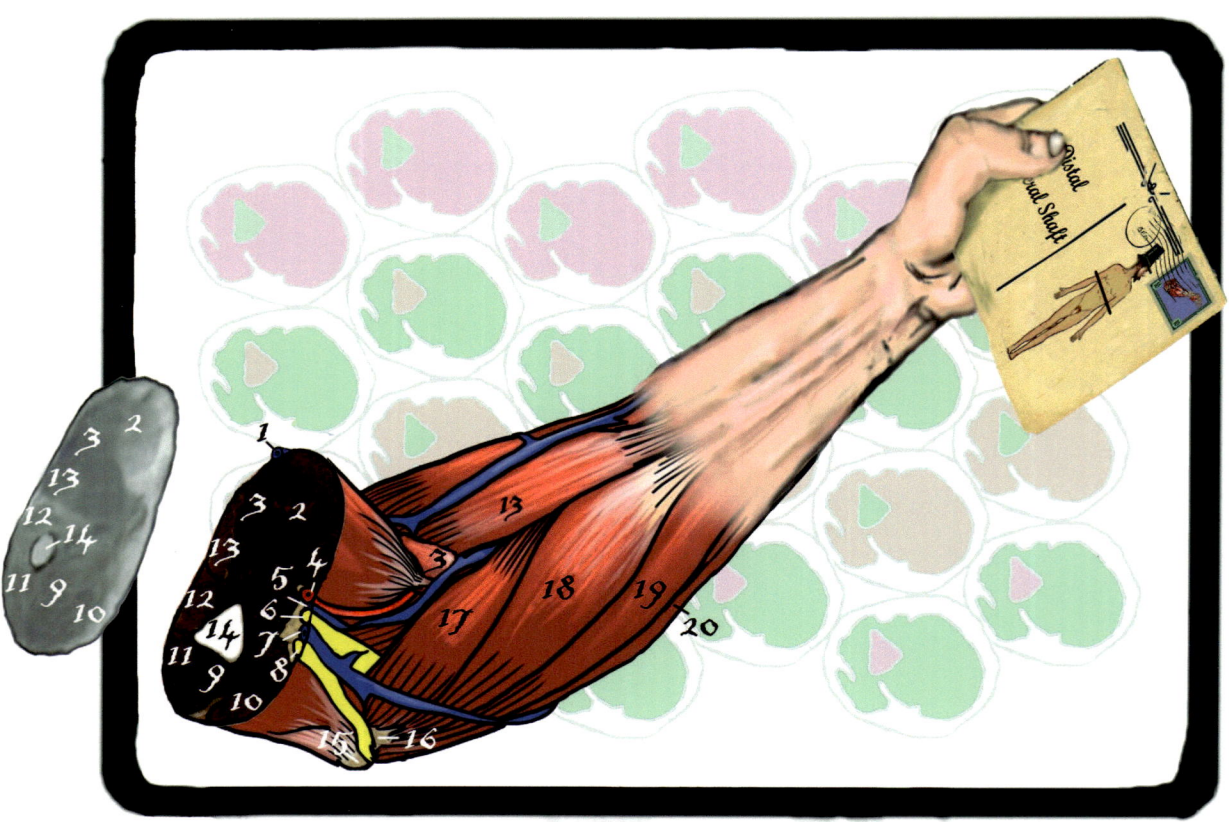

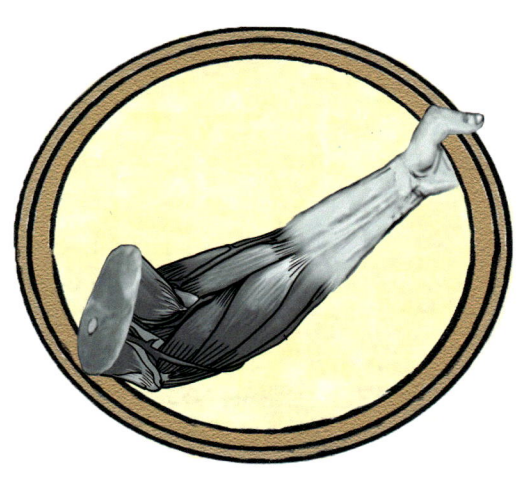

19. **Flexor digitorum superficialis** (*M. flexor digitorum superficialis*)

20. **Flexor carpi ulnaris** (M. flexor carpi ulnaris)

1.   **Cephalic vein** (*V. cephalica*)

2.   **Biceps brachii** (*M. biceps brachii*)

3.   **Brachialis** (*M. brachialis*)

4.   **Brachial artery** (*Arteria brachialis*)

5.   **Brachial vein** (*V. brachialis*)

6.   **Median nerve** (*N. medianus*)

7.   **Basilic vein** (*V. basilica*)

8.   **Ulnar nerve** (*N. ulnaris*)

9.   **Medial/deep head of the triceps** (*M. triceps brachii, caput mediale/profundus*)

10. **Long head of the triceps** (*M. triceps brachii, caput longus*)

11. **Lateral head of the triceps** (*M. triceps brachii, caput laterale*)

12. **Extensor carpi radialis longus** (*M. extensor carpi radialis longus*)

13. **Brachioradialis** (*M. brachioradialis*)

14. **Humerus** (*Humerus*)

15. **Olecranon** (*Olecranon*)

16. **Medial epicondyle of the humerus** (*Epicondylus medialis*)

17. **Pronator teres** (*M. pronator teres*)

18. **Flexor carpi radialis and palmaris longus** (*M. flexor carpi radialis et palmaris longus*)

V – Proximal Antebrachium – Extensor Surface

This cut shows the extensor structures in the proximal forearm. Extensor carpi radialis longus and brevis are seen in the 12 o'clock position, sitting just ulnar to brachioradialis. The cephalic vein spirals around the forearm radially, while the basilic vein is more ulnar. Supinator can be seen wrapping around the radius bone, as a wisp of anconeus lies against the ulna. An MR has been positioned at the same angle as the anatomic structures.

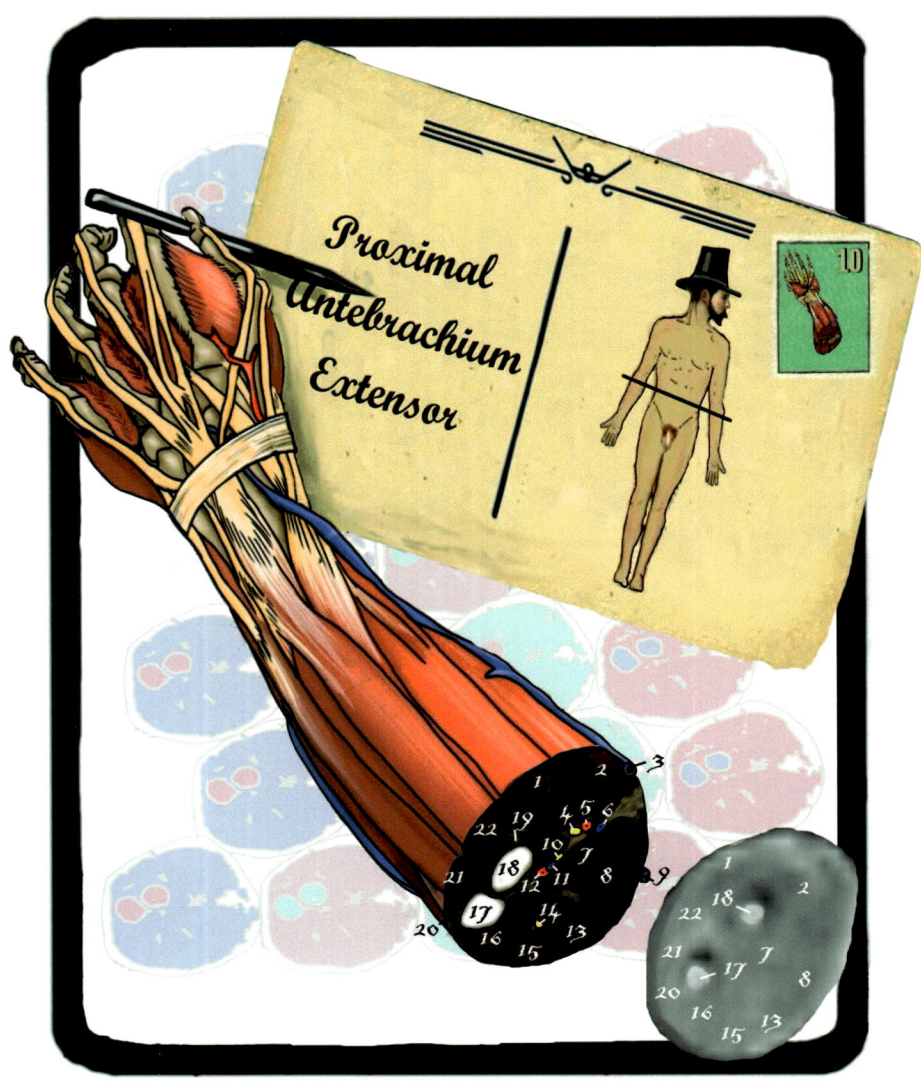

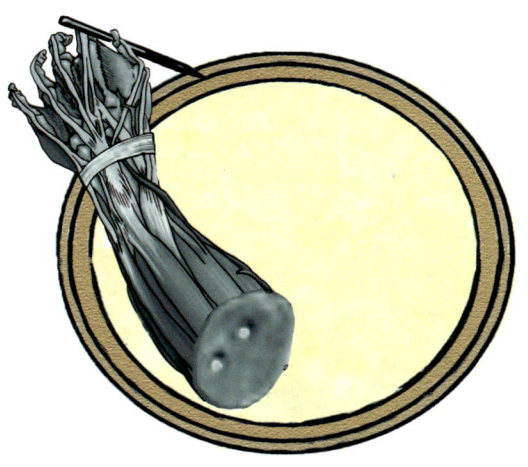

18. **Radius** (*Radius*) Derived from the Latin term for a spoke, the bone was named by Celsus in the 1st century for its resemblance to that part of a wheel.

19. **Supinator** (*M. supinator*)

20. **Anconeus** (*M. anconeus*) From the Greek term, αγκων, meaning the bend of the elbow.

21. **Extensor carpi ulnaris** (*M. extensor carpi ulnaris*)

22. **Extensor digitorum** (*M. extensor digitorum*)

1. **Extensor carpi radialis longus and brevis** (*M. extensor carpi radialis longus et brevis*)

2. **Brachioradialis** (*M. brachioradialis*)

3. **Cephalic vein** (*V. cephalica*)

4. **Radial nerve** (*N. radialis*)

5. **Radial artery** (*Arteria radialis*)

6. **Radial vein** (*Vena radialis*)

7. **Pronator teres** (*M. pronator teres*)

8. **Flexor carpi radialis** (*M. flexor carpi radialis*)

9. **Basilic vein** (*V. basilica*)

10. **Median nerve** (*N. medianus*)

11. **Ulnar vein** (*V. ulnaris*)

12. **Ulnar artery** (*Arteria ulnaris*)

13. **Flexor digitorum superficialis** (*M. flexor digitorum superficialis*)

14. **Ulnar nerve** (*N. ulnaris*)

15. **Flexor carpi ulnaris** (*M. flexor carpi ulnaris*)

16. **Flexor digitorum profundus** (*M. flexor digitorum profundus*)

17. **Ulna** (*Ulna*) From the Latin, meaning elbow, and the Greek, ωλένη. The name was first used by Celsus.

VI – Proximal Antebrachium – Flexor Surface

This section is the flexor aspect of section V, the proximal forearm. The basilic vein is in the 12 o'clock position, anterior to flexor digitorum superficialis, which lies between flexor ulnaris, and flexor carpi radialis. A sliver of pronator teres, on its way to insert onto the radius, is seen just radial to flexor carpi radialis. Supinator, again, wraps around the radius, the bulk of its belly inclined posteriorly, towards 6 o'clock. The corresponding MR has been rotated at the same angle as the anatomic structures.

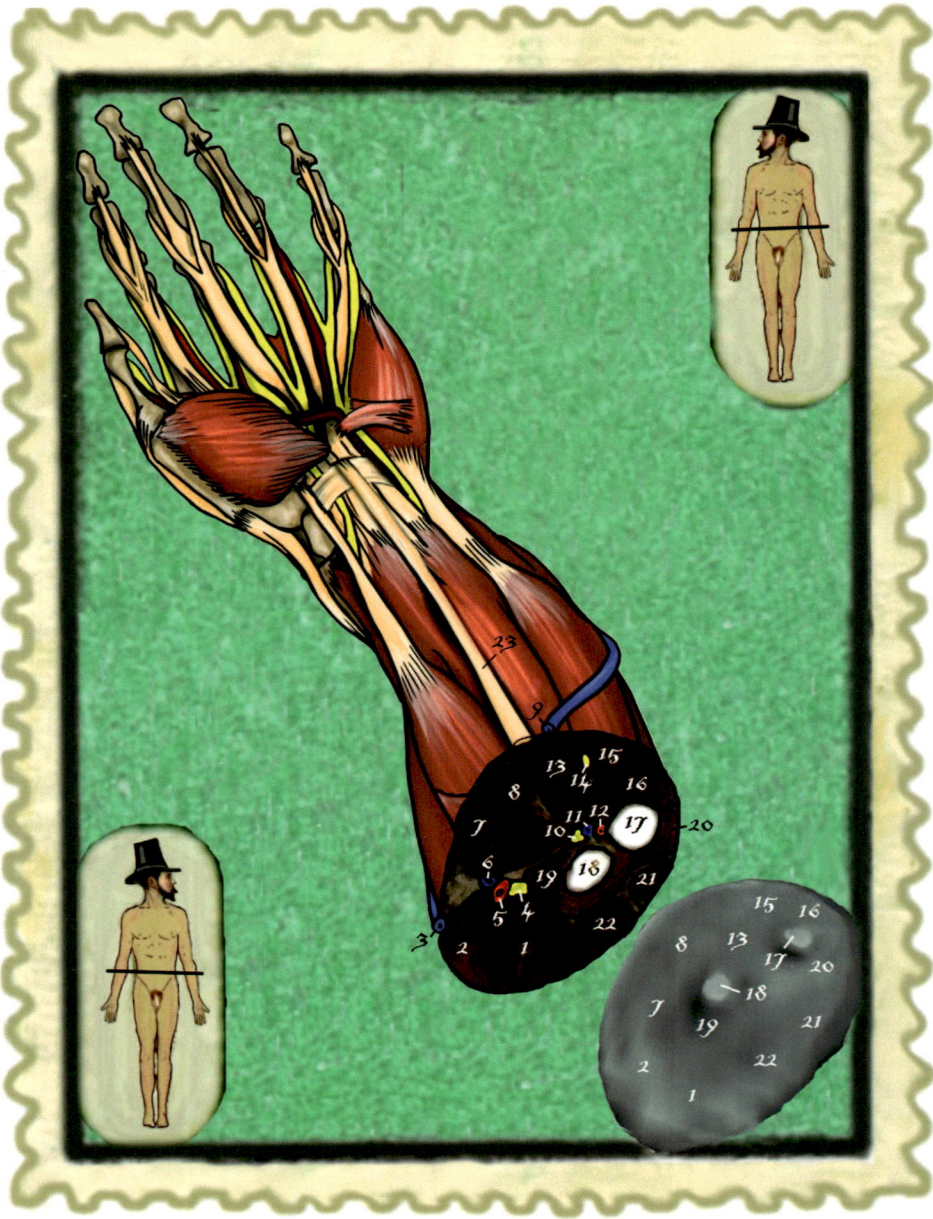

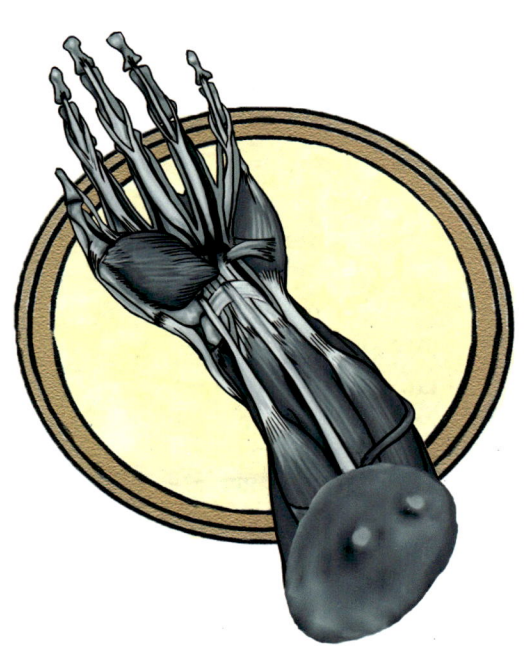

17. **Ulna** (*Ulna*)

18. **Radius** (*Radius*)

19. **Supinator** (*M. supinator*)

20. **Anconeus** (*M. anconeus*)

21. **Extensor carpi ulnaris** (*M. extensor carpi ulnaris*)

22. **Extensor digitorum** (*M. extensor digitorum*)

23. **Palmaris longus tendon** (*Ten. palmaris longus*)

1. **Extensor carpi radialis longus and brevis** (*M. extensor carpi radialis longus et brevis*)

2. **Brachioradialis** (*M. brachioradialis*)

3. **Cephalic vein** (*V. cephalica*)

4. **Radial nerve** (*N. radialis*)

5. **Radial artery** (*Arteria radialis*)

6. **Radial vein** (*Vena radialis*)

7. **Pronator teres** (*M. pronator teres*)

8. **Flexor carpi radialis** (*M. flexor carpi radialis*)

9. **Basilic vein** (*V. basilica*)

10. **Median nerve** (*N. medianus*)

11. **Ulnar vein** (*V. ulnaris*)

12. **Ulnar artery** (*Arteria ulnaris*)

13. **Flexor digitorum superficialis** (*M. flexor digitorum superficialis*)

14. **Ulnar nerve** (*N. ulnaris*)

15. **Flexor carpi ulnaris** (*M. flexor carpi ulnaris*)

16. **Flexor digitorum profundus** (*M. flexor digitorum profundus*)

VII – Distal Antebrachium – Extensor Surface

This section is of the extensor structures in the distal forearm. Extensor pollicis brevis and abductor pollicis longus are here becoming tendinous, and once seen in cross- section, these tendons can be traced distally. Extensor carpi radialis brevis and longus can likewise be traced from muscles seen radially out to their distal tendons. On the ulnar side, flexor carpi ulnaris, sitting adjacent to the ulna, begins to become more tendinous, as are its neighbors, extensor digiti minimi, extensor pollicis longus, and extensor digitorum. An MR corresponds.

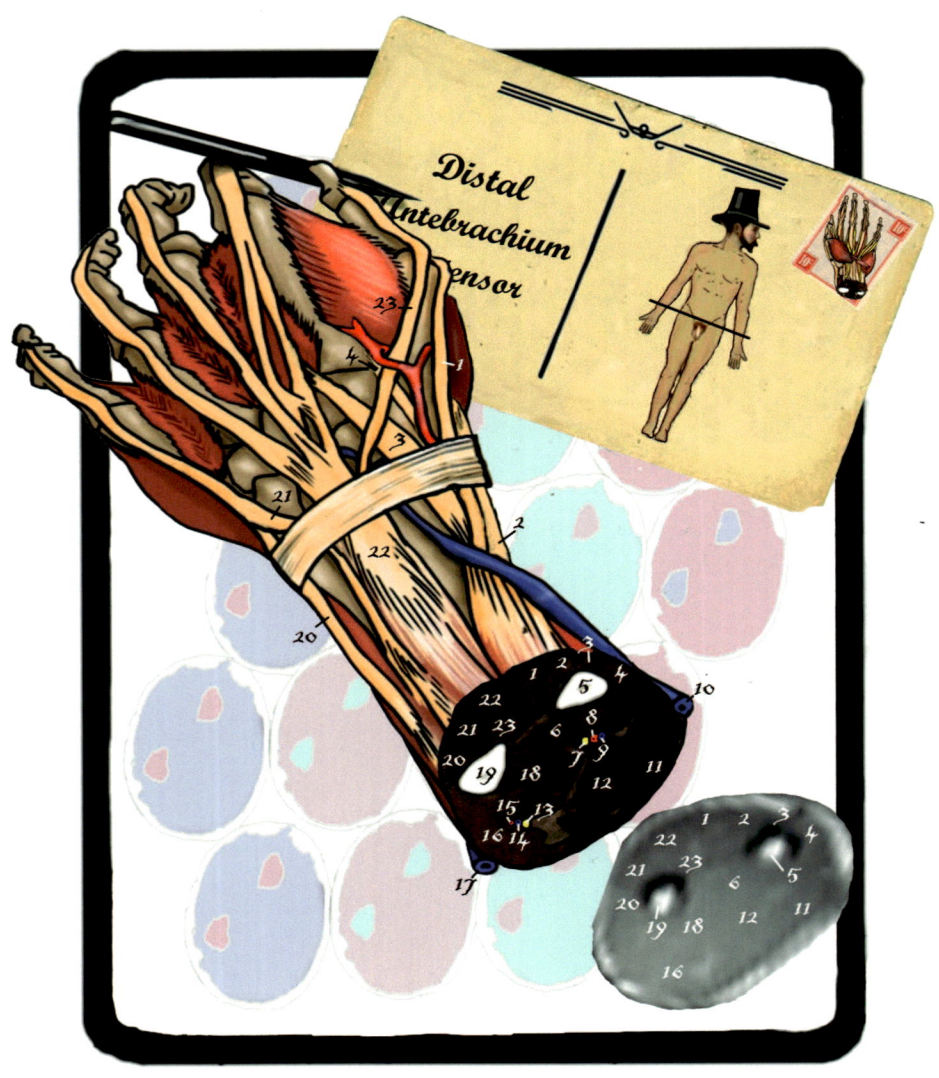

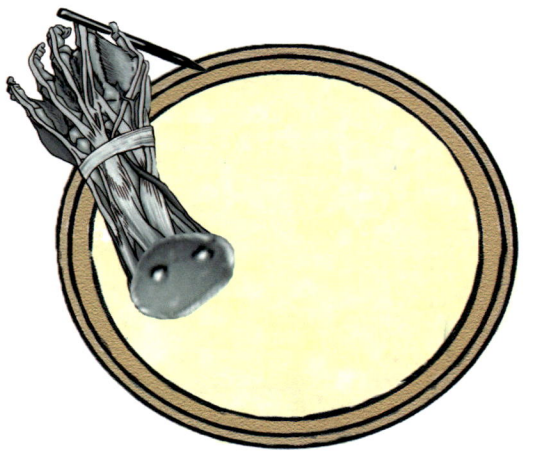

17. **Basilic vein** (*V. basilica*)

18. **Flexor digitorum profundus** (*M. flexor digitorum profundus*)

19. **Ulna** (*Ulna*)

20. **Extensor carpi ulnaris muscle and tendon** (*M. et ten. extensor carpi ulnaris*)

21. **Extensor digiti minimi muscle and tendon** (*M. et ten. extensor digiti minimi*) The term minimi is derived from the Latin word minimus, which means tiny.

22. **Extensor digitorum muscle and tendon** (*M. et ten. extensor digitorum*)

23. **Extensor pollicis longus muscle and tendon** (*M. et ten. extensor pollicis longus*)

1. **Extensor pollicis brevis muscle and tendon** (*M. et ten. extensor pollicis brevis*)

2. **Abductor pollicis longus muscle and tendon** (*M. et ten. abductor pollicis longus*)

3. **Extensor carpi radialis brevis muscle and tendon** (*M. et ten. extensor carpi radialis brevis*)

4. **Extensor carpi radialis longus muscle and tendon** (*M. et ten. extensor carpi radialis longus*)

5. **Radius** (*Radius*)

6. **Flexor pollicis longus** (*M. flexor pollicis longus*)

7. **Median nerve** (*N. medianus*)

8. **Radial artery** (*Arteria radialis*)

9. **Radial vein** (*Vena radialis*)

10. **Cephalic vein** (*V. cephalica*)

11. **Flexor carpi radialis** (*M. flexor carpi radialis*)

12. **Flexor digitorum superficialis** (*M. flexor digitorum superficialis*)

13. **Ulnar nerve** (*N. ulnaris*)

14. **Ulnar vein** (*V. ulnaris*)

15. **Ulnar artery** (*Arteria ulnaris*)

16. **Flexor carpi ulnaris** (*M. flexor carpi ulnaris*)

VIII – Distal Antebrachium – Flexor Surface

A slice through the distal forearm shows the flexor compartment. The tendons of flexor digitorum superficialis are seen in the 12 o'clock position, their muscle bellies lying more posterior. Flexor carpi ulnaris is becoming less muscle belly and more tendon, and its distal insertion on the base of the fifth metacarpal and pisiform can be appreciated. Pronator quadratus sits between the radius and the ulna, while posterior to the ulna, at 7 o'clock, extensor tendons can be seen, structures best appreciated when juxtaposed with VII. The corresponding MR is shown.

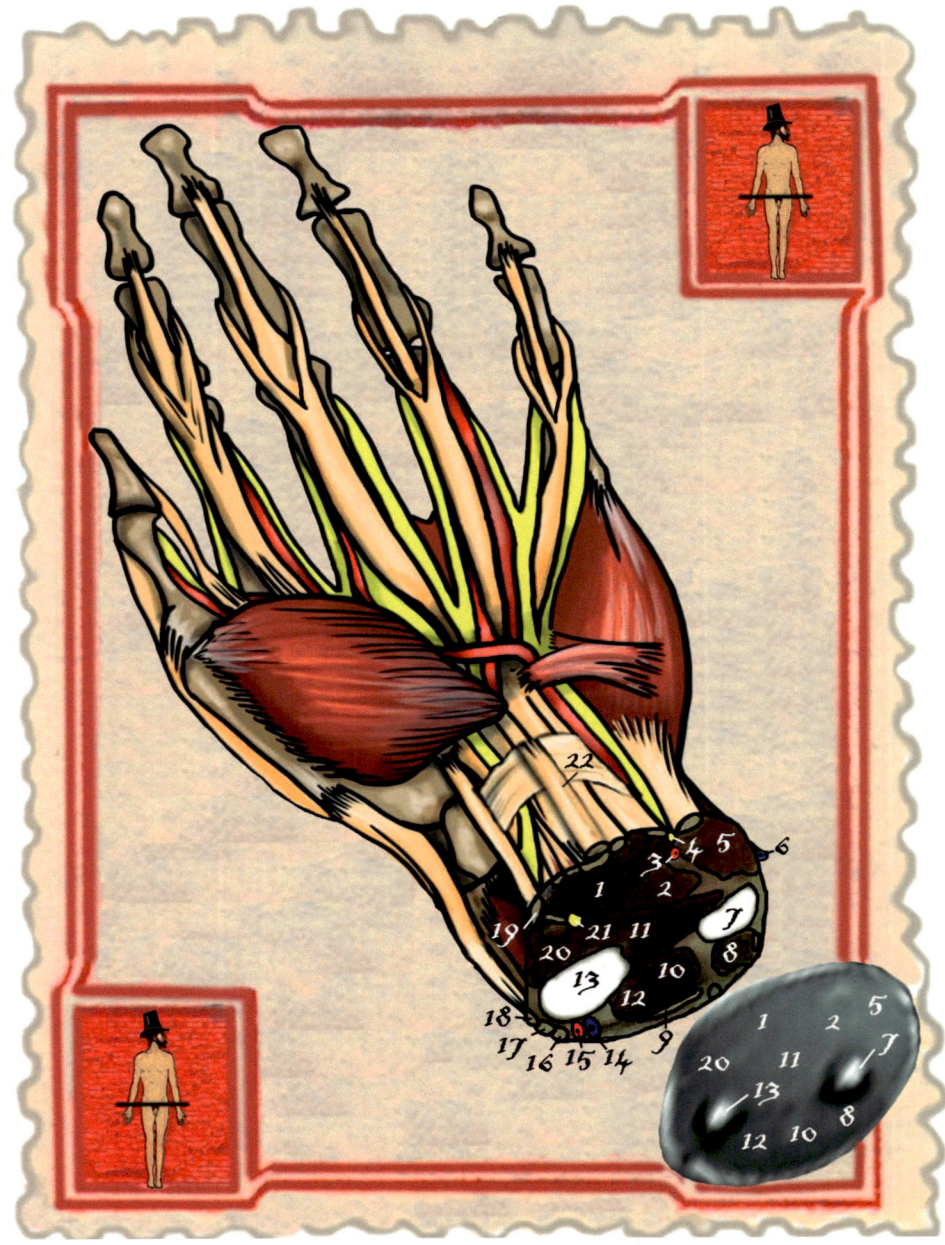

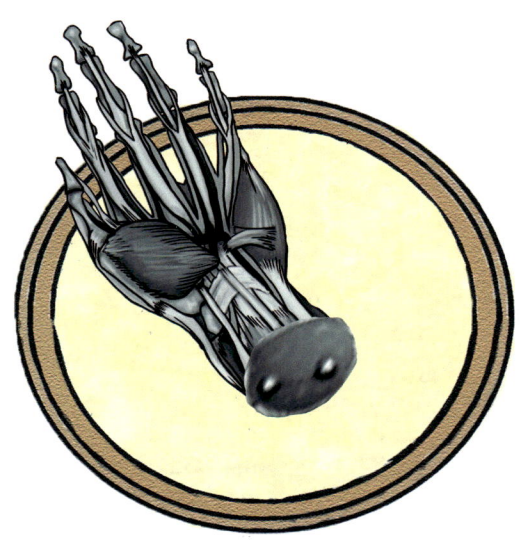

16. **Extensor pollicis brevis tendon** (*Ten. extensor pollicis brevis*)

17. **Extensor carpi radialis longus and brevis tendon** (*Ten. extensor carpi radialis longus et brevis*)

18. **Abductor pollicis longus tendon** (*Ten. abductor pollicis longus*)

19. **Flexor carpi radialis tendon** (*Ten. flexor carpi radialis*)

20. **Flexor pollicis longus muscle and tendon** (*M. et ten. flexor pollicis longus*)

21. **Median nerve** (*N. medianus*)

22. **Palmaris longus tendon** (*Ten. palmaris longus*)

1. **Flexor digitorum superficialis muscle and tendon** (*M. et ten. flexor digitorum superficialis*)

2. **Flexor digitorum profundus** (*M. flexor digitorum profundus*)

3. **Ulnar artery** (*Arteria ulnaris*)

4. **Ulnar nerve** (*N. ulnaris*)

5. **Flexor carpi ulnaris muscle and tendon** (*M. et ten. flexor carpi ulnaris*)

6. **Basilic vein** (*V. basilica*)

7. **Ulna** (*Ulna*)

8. **Extensor carpi ulnaris muscle and tendon** (*M. et ten. extensor carpi ulnaris*)

9. **Extensor digitorum tendon** (*Ten. extensor digitorum*)

10. **Extensor indicis** (*M. extensor indicis*)

11. **Pronator quadratus** (*M. pronator quadratus*)

12. **Extensor pollicis longus muscle** (*M. extensor pollicis longus*)

13. **Radius** (*Radius*)

14. **Cephalic vein** (*V. cephalica*)

15. **Radial artery** (*Arteria radialis*)

IX – Proximal Carpal Row – Flexor Surface

This section is of the proximal carpal row, and highlights the flexor compartment. The term carpus, from κορπός, was first used by Galen to describe the bones of the wrist. The flexor retinaculum, which spans the wrist like a bow string, has been removed so as to better visualize the contents of the carpal tunnel. The tendons of the flexors digitorum and pollicis longus are seen within the curvature of the carpal bones, along with the median nerve. As the corresponding radiographic studies from the Visible Human were too distorted and oblique, an idealized CT was re-created for this section, emphasizing the proximal row of carpal bones.

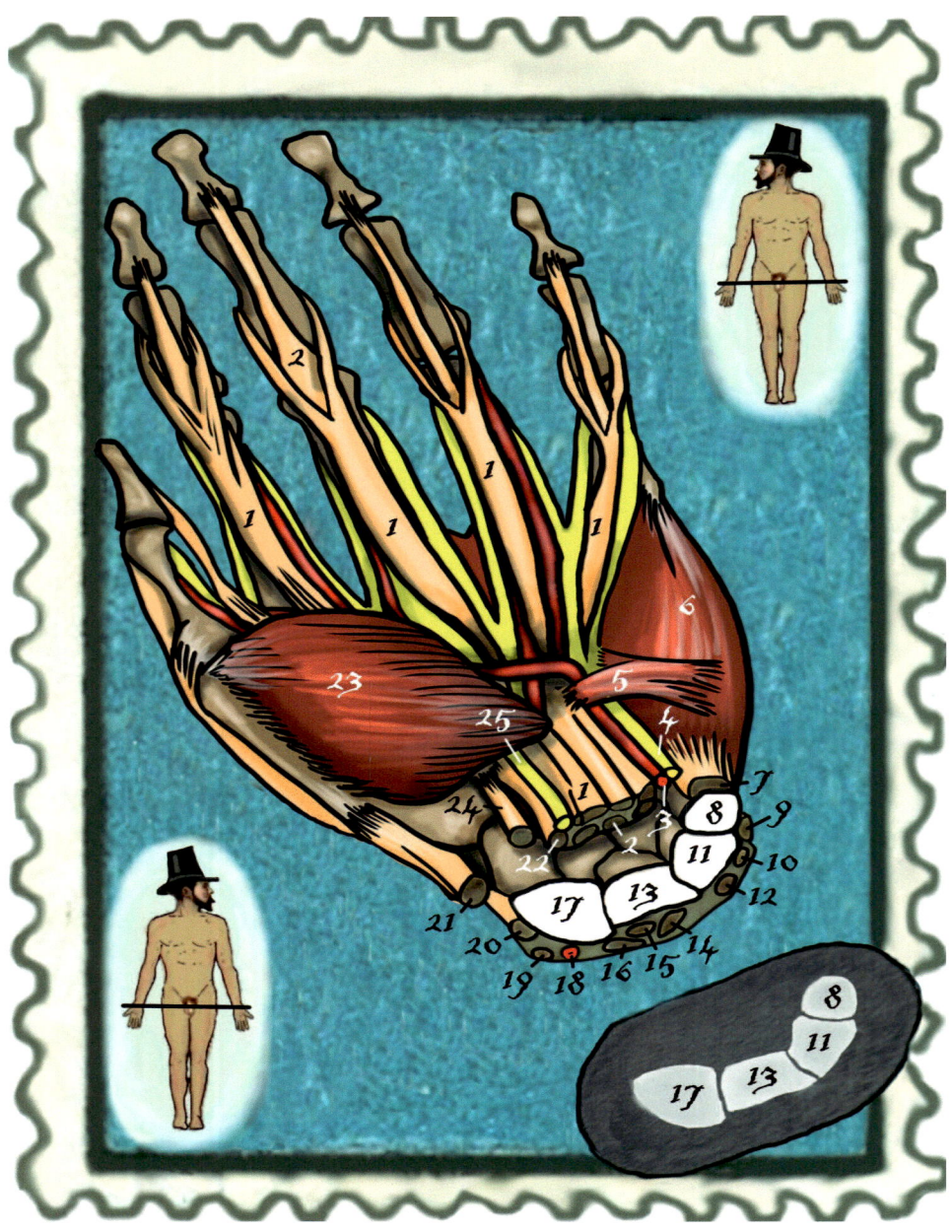

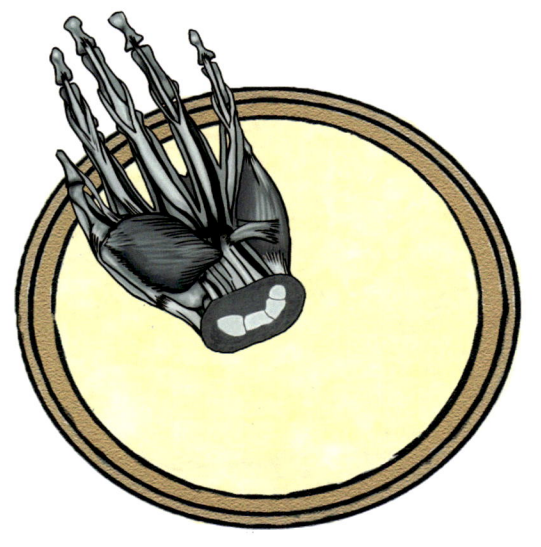

1. **Flexor digitorum superficialis tendon** (*Ten. flexor digitorum superficialis*)

2. **Flexor digitorum profundus tendon** (*Ten. flexor digitorum profundus*)

3. **Ulnar artery** (*Arteria ulnaris*)

4. **Ulnar nerve** (*N. ulnaris*)

5. **Palmaris brevis** (*M. palmaris brevis*) Named by Giambattista Canano in the 16th century.

6. **Muscles of the hypothenar eminence** (*Eminentia hypothenaris*) The term was applied to the little finger by Riolan in the 17th century.

7. **Flexor carpi ulnaris tendon** (*Ten. flexor carpi ulnaris*)

8. **Pisiform** (*Os pisiforme*) From the Latin pisa, meaning pea: the pisiform is pea-like.

9. **Extensor carpi ulnaris tendon** (*Ten. extensor carpi ulnaris*)

10. **Extensor digiti minimi muscle and tendon** (*M. et ten. extensor digiti minimi*)

11. **Triquetrum** (*Os triquetrum*) From the Latin, triquetrus, meaning three-sided.

12. **Extensor digitorum tendon** (*Ten. extensor digitorum*)

13. **Lunate** (*Os lunatum*) From the Latin luna, meaning moon, due to its resemblance of a crescent moon on profile.

14. **Extensor indicis tendon** (*Ten. extensor indicis*)

15. **Extensor carpi radialis brevis tendon** (*Ten. extensor carpi radialis brevis*)

16. **Extensor pollicis longus tendon** (*Ten. extensor pollicis longus*)

17. **Scaphoid** (*Os scaphoideum*) From, σκαφη, meaning hollowed out, and so named for its concave faces that accommodate other bones.

18. **Radial artery** (*Arteria radialis*)

19. **Extensor carpi radialis longus tendon** (*Ten. extensor carpi radialis longus*)

20. **Extensor pollicis brevis tendon** (*Ten. extensor pollicis brevis*)

21. **Abductor pollicis longus tendon** (*Ten. abductor pollicis longus*)

22. **Flexor pollicis longus tendon** (*Ten. flexor pollicis longus*)

23. **Muscles of the thenar eminence** (*Eminentia thenaris*) Derived from θέναρ, meaning the flat of the hand, the term was applied to the thumb by Riolan in the 17th century.

24. **Flexor carpi radialis tendon** (*Ten. flexor carpi radialis*)

25. **Median nerve** (*(N. medianus)*)

X – Distal Carpal Row – Extensor Surface

This section is a replanarized cut through the distal row of the carpus and shows the extensor surface. At 12 o'clock sit the tendons of extensor digitorum, and just radial to this is the tendon of extensor indicis. The distal row of the carpal bones are arched like a taut bow, and within the hollow of the carpal tunnel the tendons of the flexors digitorum, pollicis longus, and the median nerve move beneath an imagined bow string to their distal destinations. The flexor retinaculum has been removed. As the corresponding radiographic studies from the Visible Human were too distorted and oblique, an idealized CT was created for the section emphasizing the distal row of carpal bones.

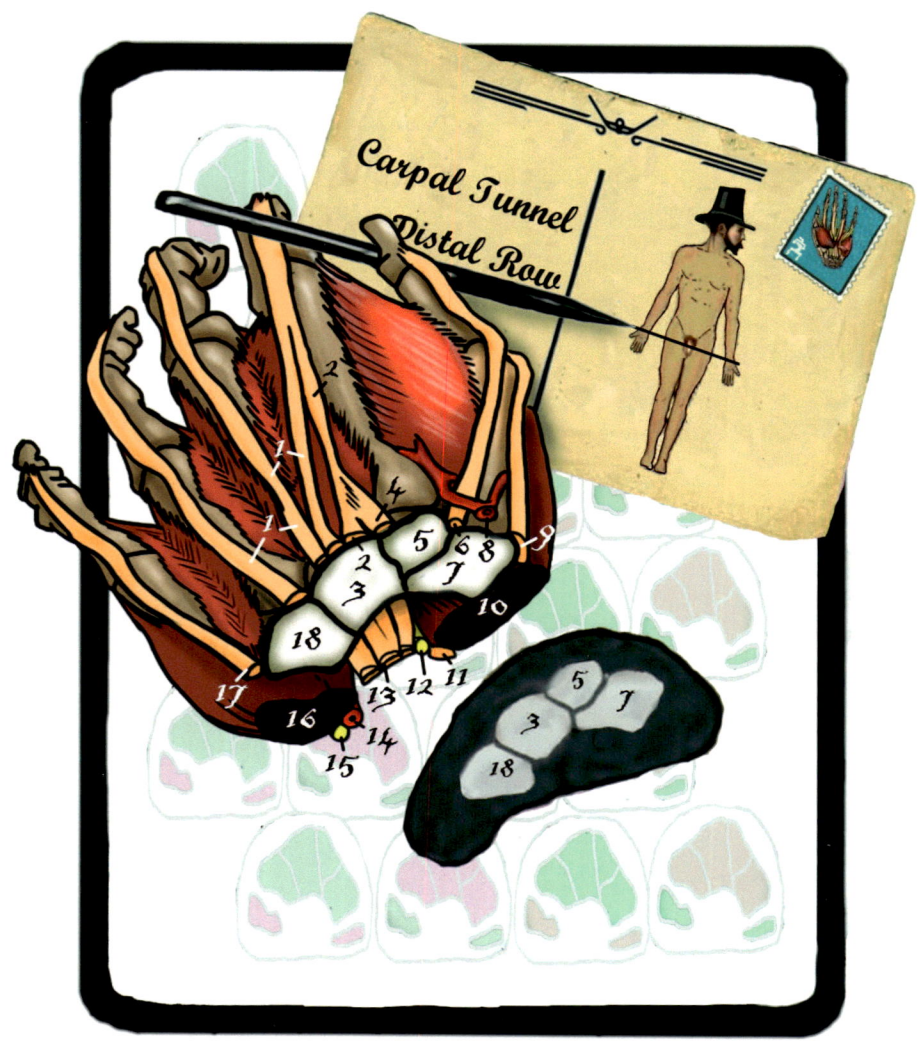

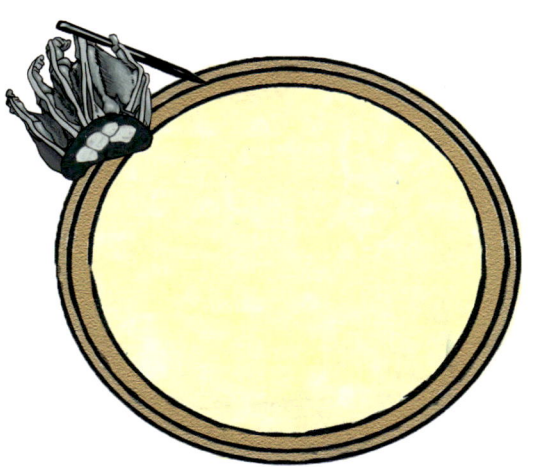

15. **Ulnar nerve** (*N. ulnaris*)

16. **Muscles of the hypothenar eminence** (*Eminentia hypothenaris*)

17. **Extensor digiti minimi tendon** (*Ten. extensor digiti minimi*)

18. **Hamate** (*Os hamatum*) From the Latin term hamatus, meaning hooked.

1. **Extensor digitorum tendon** (*Ten. extensor digitorum*)

2. **Extensor indicis tendon** (*Ten. extensor indicis*)

3. **Capitate** (*Os capitatum*) Derived from the Latin, caput, meaning not only head but also a smooth, rounded structure.

4. **Extensor carpi radialis brevis tendon** (*Ten. extensor carpi radialis brevis*)

5. **Trapezoid** (*Os trapezoideum*)

6. **Extensor pollicis longus tendon** (*Ten. extensor pollicis longus*)

7. **Trapezium** (*Os trapezium*) From τραπέζιου, a small table.

8. **Radial artery** (*Arteria radialis*)

9. **Extensor pollicis brevis tendon** (*Ten. extensor pollicis brevis*)

10. **Muscles of the thenar eminence** (*Eminentia thenaris*)

11. **Flexor pollicis longus tendon** (*Ten. flexor pollicis longus*)

12. **Median nerve** (*N. medianus*)

13. **Flexor digitorum superficialis and profundus tendon** (*Ten. flexor digitorum superficialis et profundus*)

14. **Ulnar artery** (*Arteria ulnaris*)

XI – Mid – Metacarpal – Flexor Surface

Here the hand has been sectioned and replanarized through the middle of the metacarpal shaft. The tendon of flexor pollicis longus is seen surrounded by the muscles of the thenar eminence. The tendons of the flexors digitorum are surrounded by the lumbricals, and their distal courses can be traced from the axial plane, up to the superficialis' bifurcation of Camper's chiasm, a passage that allows profundus a clear path to the distal phalanx. The digital branches of the median and ulnar nerve can also be traced from the cross-section to their respective points of distal innervation. The corresponding MR is cut obliquely, thus making the thenar muscles appear less prominent than the hypothenar muscles.

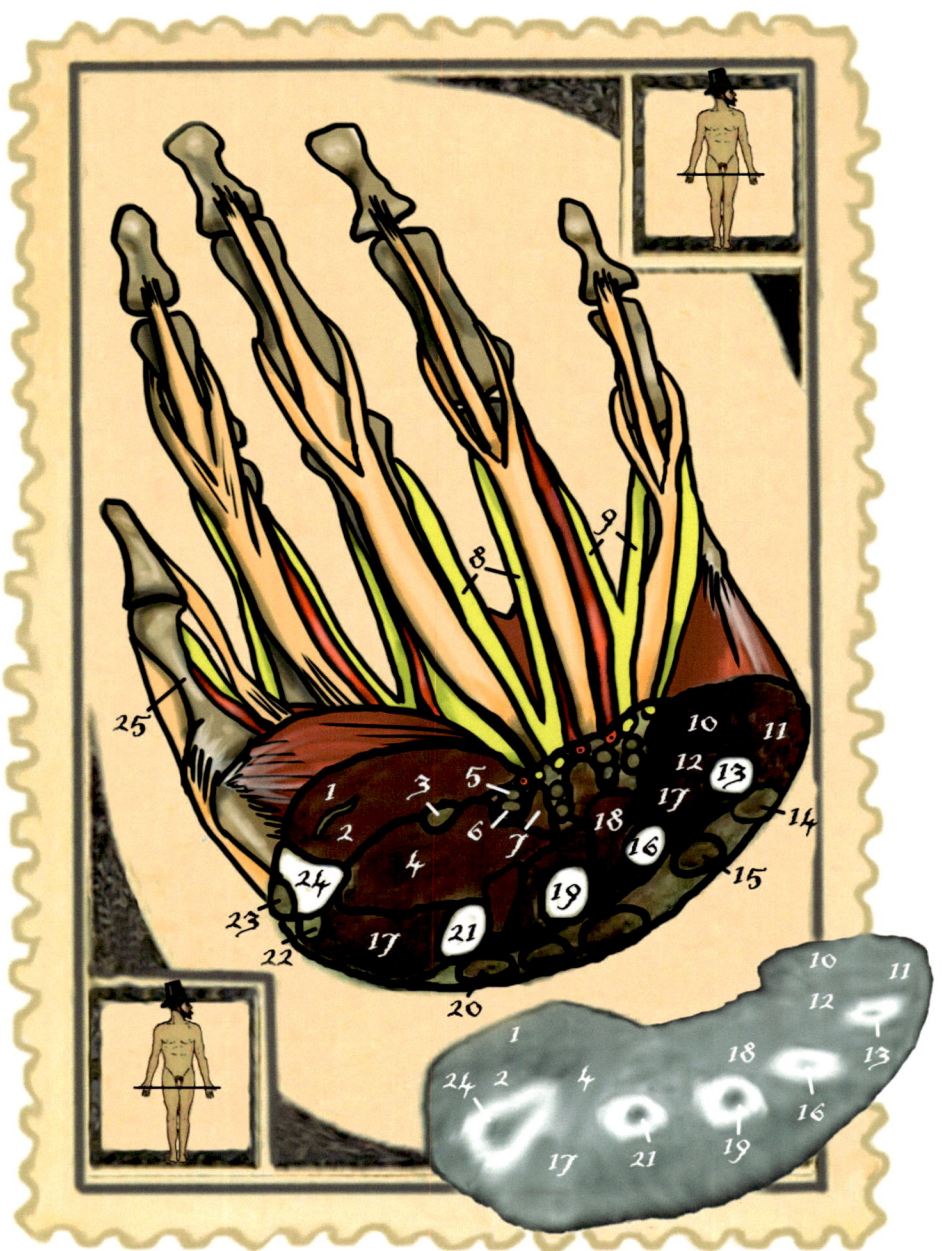

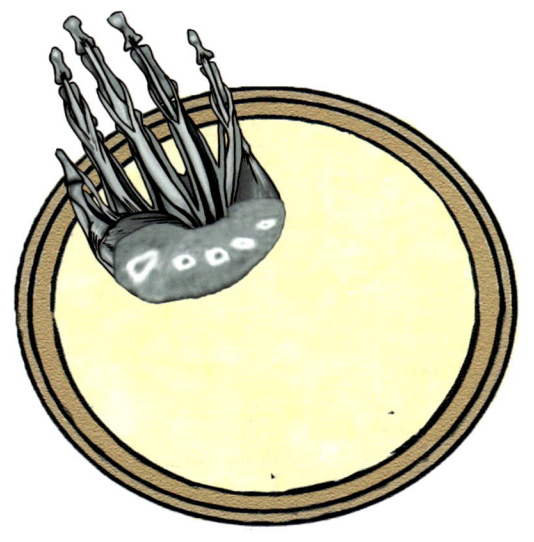

1. **Abductor pollicis** (*M. abductor pollicis*)

2. **Flexor pollicis brevis** (*M. flexor pollicis brevis*)

3. **Flexor pollicis longus tendon** (*Ten. flexor pollicis longus*)

4. **Adductor pollicis** (*M. adductor pollicis*)

5. **Flexor digitorum superficialis tendon** (*Ten. flexor digitorum superficialis*)

6. **Flexor digitorum profundus tendon** (*Ten. flexor digitorum profundus*)

7. **Lumbricals** (*Mm. lumbricales*) Derived from the Latin term lumbricus, meaning worm, the muscles were named by Riolan.

8. **Proper palmar digital branches of the median nerve** (*N. medianus, Nn. Digitales palmares proprii*)

9. **Proper palmar digital branches of the ulnar nerve** (*N. ulnaris, Nn. Digitales palmares proprii*)

10. **Flexor digiti minimi** (*M. flexor digiti minimi*)

11. **Abductor digiti minimi** (*M. abductor digiti minimi*)

12. **Opponens digiti minimi** (*M. opponens digiti minimi*)

13. **Body of the fifth metacarpal** (*Corpus ossis metacarpi V*)

14. **Extensor digiti minimi tendon** (*Ten. extensor digiti minimi*)

15. **Extensor digitorum tendon** (*Ten. extensor digitorum*)

16. **Body of the fourth metacarpal** (*Corpus ossis metacarpi IV*)

17. **Dorsal interossei** (*Mm. interossei dorsales*)

18. **Palmar interossei** (*Mm. interossei palmares*)

19. **Body of the third metacarpal** (*Corpus ossis metacarpi III*)

20. **Extensor indicis tendon** (*Ten. extensor indicis*)

21. **Body of the second metacarpal** (*Corpus ossis metacarpi II*)

22. **Extensor pollicis longus tendon** (*Ten. extensor pollicis longus*)

23. **Extensor pollicis brevis tendon** (*Ten. extensor pollicis brevis*)

24. **Body of the first metacarpal** (*Corpus ossis metacarpi II*)

25. **Proximal phalanx** (*Phalanx proximalis*) Derived from φάλαγξ, meaning line of battle, the name was given by Aristotle.

Part 2:
The Lower Extremity

I – Superior Femoral Diaphysis – Medial

In this section the leg has been sliced through the superior thigh, and rotated to show its medial surface. Rectus femoris is seen at the 12 o'clock position. Medial to r. femoris is sartorius, whose meandering body can be followed down to the tendons of pes-anserinus (goose's foot) near the knee. The relation of thigh muscles to the adductor group can be appreciated in this section. Sartorius lies above vastus medialis, and adductor longus, in the 2 o'clock position, is seen ducking beneath both of these muscles. At 3 o'clock is gracilis, sitting above adductor magnus. The medial face of semimembranosus can be seen at 6 o'clock. A corresponding CT shows these structures radiographically.

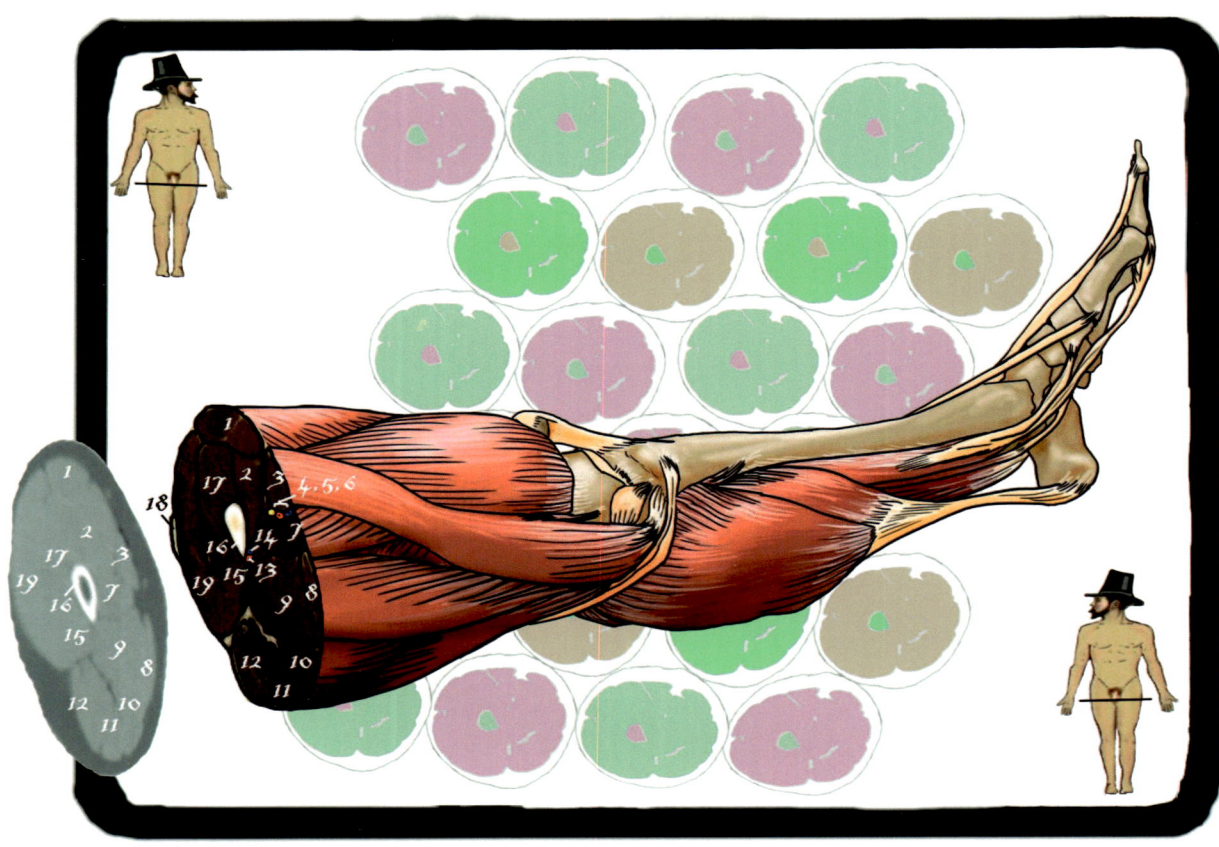

15. **Short head of biceps femoris** (*M. biceps femoris, caput breve*)

16. **Shaft of the femur** (*Corpus femoris*) Latin for thigh. Singer writes that the term may be related to the verb fero, meaning I bear, or feo, the root of the term foetus, suggesting the relationship between the thighs and bearing children.

17. **Vastus intermedius** (*M. vastus intermedius*)

18. **Iliotibial tract** (*Tractus iliotibialis*)

19. **Vastus lateralis** (*M. vastus lateralis*)

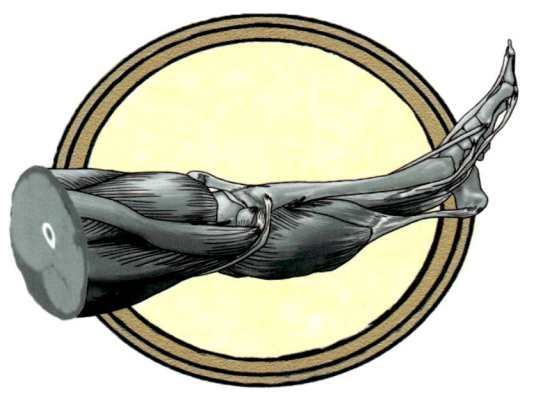

1. **Rectus femoris** (*M. rectus femoris*)

2. **Vastus medialis** (*M. vastus medialis*) The term vastus, meaning large in Latin, was given to thigh muscles by Riolan, a 17th century anatomist.

3. **Sartorius** (*M. sartorius*) Derived from the Latin, sartor, meaning a tailor, the muscle was named by Spigelius, a 17th century Belgian anatomist.

4. **Femoral vein** (*V. femoralis*)

5. **Femoral artery** (*A. femoralis*)

6. **Femoral nerve** (*N. femoralis*)

7. **Adductor longus** (*M. adductor longus*)

8. **Gracilis** (*M. gracilis*) Latin for slender, the muscle was named by Douglas, an 18th century anatomist.

9. **Adductor magnus** (*M. adductor magnus*)

10. **Semimembranosus** (*M. semimembranosus*)

11. **Semitendinosus** (*M. semitendinosus*)

12. **Long head of biceps femoris** (*M. biceps femoris, caput longum*) The biceps femoris were named by Bartholin in the 18th century.

13. **Profunda femoris vein** (*Vena profunda femoris*)

14. **Profunda femoris artery** (*Arteria profunda femoris*)

II – Superior Femoral Diaphysis – Lateral

In this section the superior aspect of the femoral diaphysis has been sliced and rotated to show lateral structures. Lateral to rectus femoris sits vastus lateralis. Beneath this muscle is vastus intermedius. Posteriorly, at the 7 o'clock position, the long head of biceps femoris is seen, while closer to the posterior aspect of the femur is the short head of biceps. A corresponding CT shows these structures radiographically.

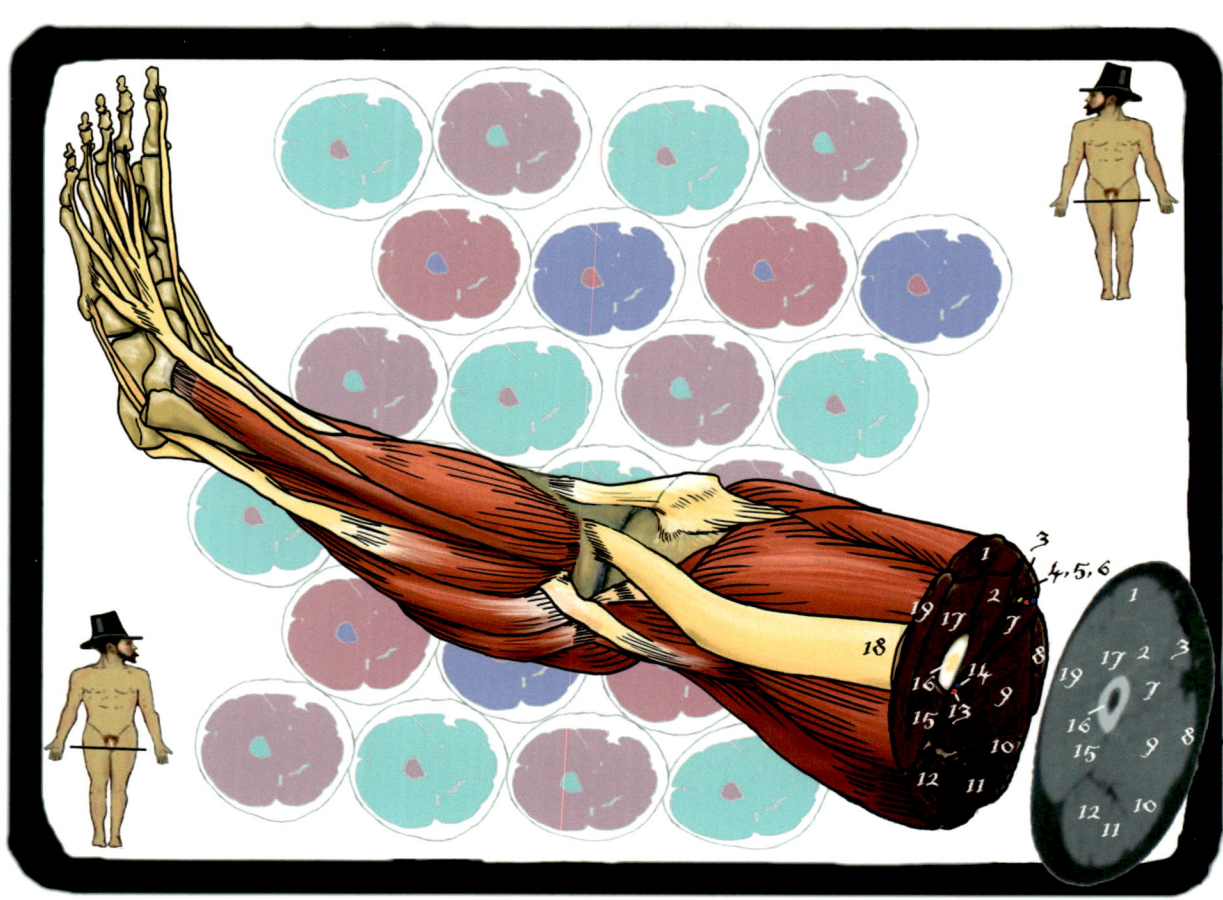

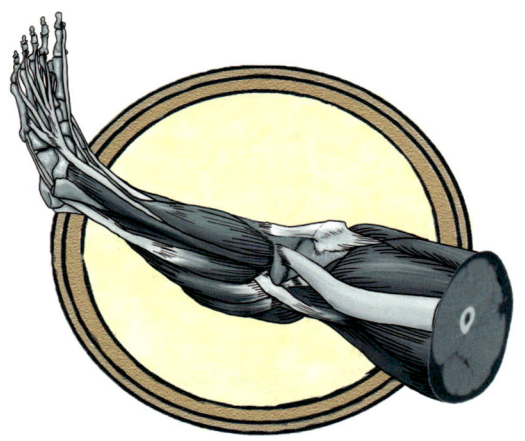

15. **Short head of biceps femoris** (*M. biceps femoris, caput breve*)

16. **Shaft of the femur** (*Corpus femoris*)

17. **Vastus intermedius** (*M. vastus intermedius*)

18. **Iliotibial tract** (*Tractus iliotibialis*)

19. **Vastus lateralis** (*M. vastus lateralis*)

1. **Rectus femoris** (*M. rectus femoris*)

2. **Vastus medialis** (*M. vastus medialis*)

3. **Sartorius** (*M. sartorius*)

4. **Femoral vein** (*V. femoralis*)

5. **Femoral artery** (*A. femoralis*)

6. **Femoral nerve** (*N. femoralis*)

7. **Adductor longus** (*M. adductor longus*)

8. **Gracilis** (*M. gracilis*)

9. **Adductor magnus** (*M. adductor magnus*)

10. **Semimembranosus** (*M. semimembranosus*)

11. **Semitendinosus** (*M. semitendinosus*)

12. **Long head of biceps femoris** (*M. biceps femoris, caput longum*)

13. **Profunda femoris artery** (*Arteria profunda femoris*)

14. **Profunda femoris vein** (*Vena profunda femoris*)

III – Superior Knee – Medial

The lower extremity has been sectioned through the superior aspect of the knee. At the 12 o'clock position, the patella and its tendon may be seen. This small bone rests above the pre-patellar bursa. At the 1 o'clock position, the fleshy part of vastus medialis is reaching its distal end. A corresponding CT shows these structures radiographically.

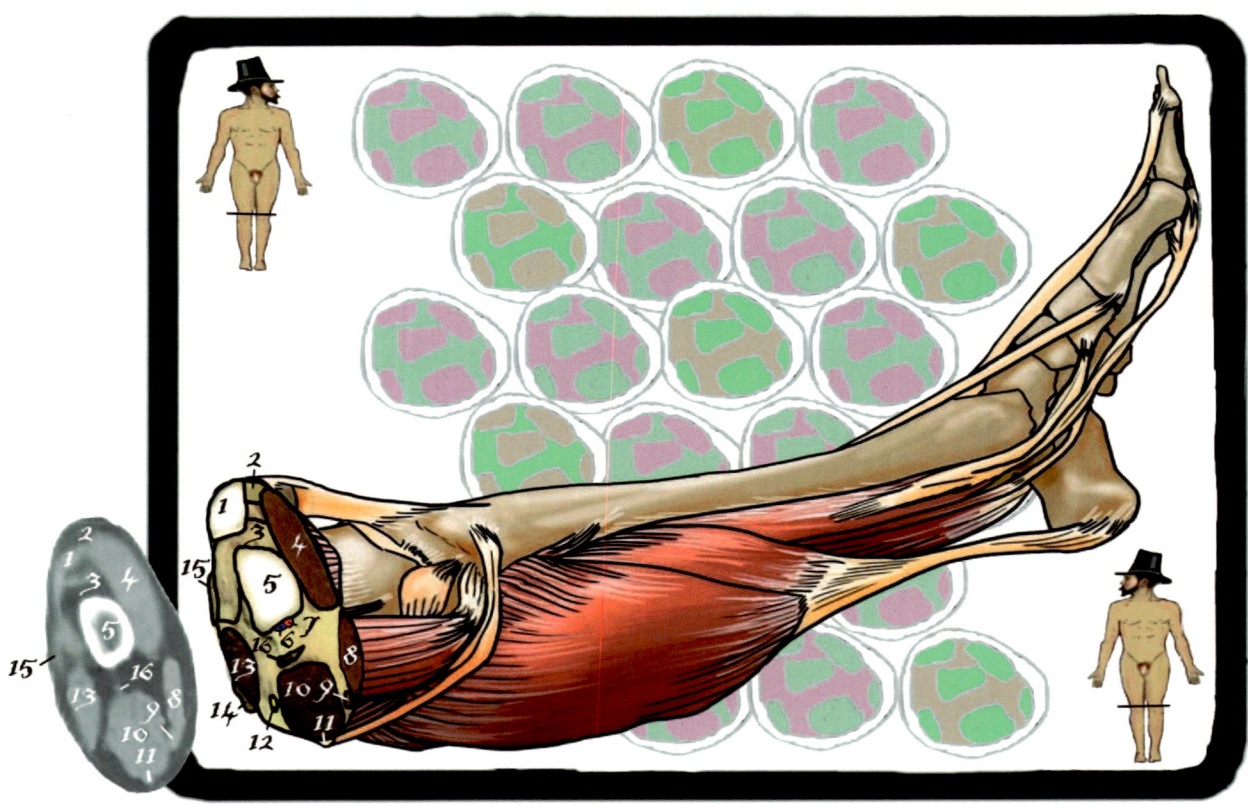

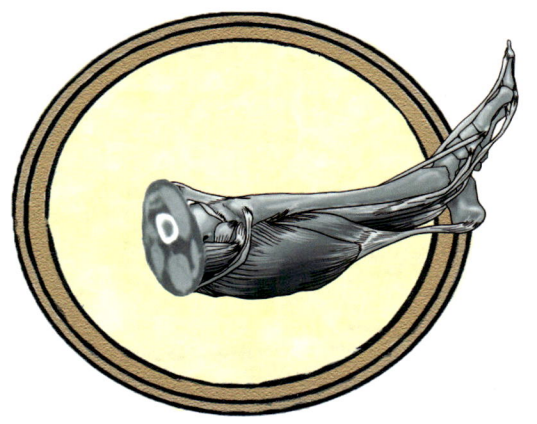

1. **Patella** (*Patella*) Latin for a small dish, or saucer, the bone was named by Celsus in the 1st century.

2. **Patellar tendon** (*Ten. patellae*)

3. **Pre-patellar bursa** (*Bursa subfascialis pre-patellaris*)

4. **Vastus medialis** (*M. vastus medialis*)

5. **Femur** (*Os femoris*)

6. **Popliteal vein** (*Vena poplitea*) The term popliteal is a derivative of the Latin term for the back of the knee, and the vessels were named by Sylvius, a 17th century French anatomist.

7. **Popliteal artery** (*Arteria poplitea*)

8. **Sartorius** (*M. sartorius*)

9. **Gracilis** (*M. gracilis*)

10. **Semimembranosus** (*M. semimembranosus*)

11. **Semitendinosus tendon** (*Ten. semitendinosus*)

12. **Tibial nerve** (*N. tibialis*)

13. **Biceps femoris** (*M. biceps femoris*)

14. **Tendon of the short head of biceps femoris** (*Ten. biceps femoris, caput breve*)

15. **Iliotibial tract** (*Tractus iliotibialis*)

16. **Lateral head of the gastrocnemius** (*M. gastrocnemius caput laterale*)

IV – Superior Knee – Lateral

In this section, the lower extremity has been sliced at the superior knee, and rotated to show lateral structures. The pre-patella bursa, sitting superior to the femur, is seen wrapping itself laterally. At 9 o'clock, the iliotibial tract tapers off to the lower leg. At 8 o'clock, the belly of biceps femoris is tapering off to a tendon. Semimembranosus sits at 6 o'clock. A corresponding CT shows these structures radiographically.

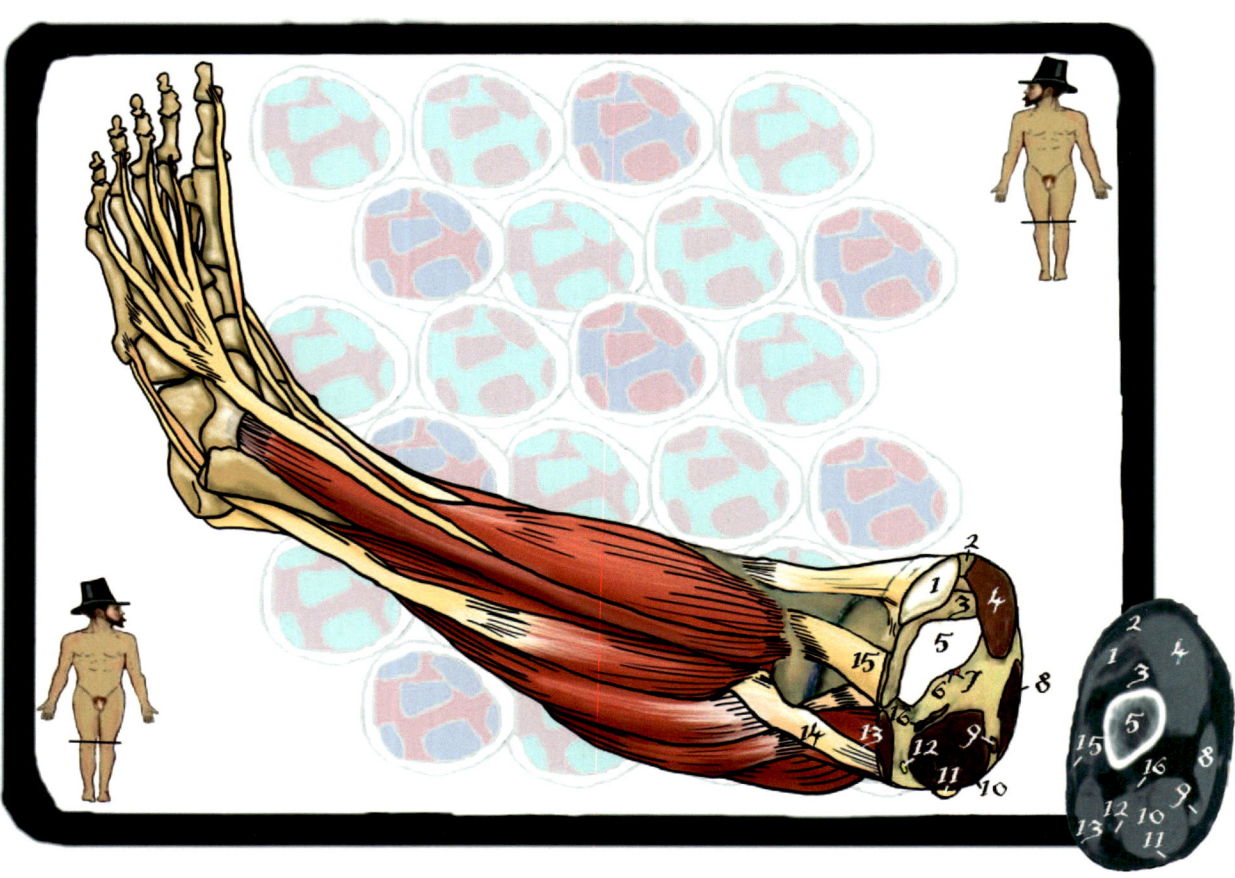

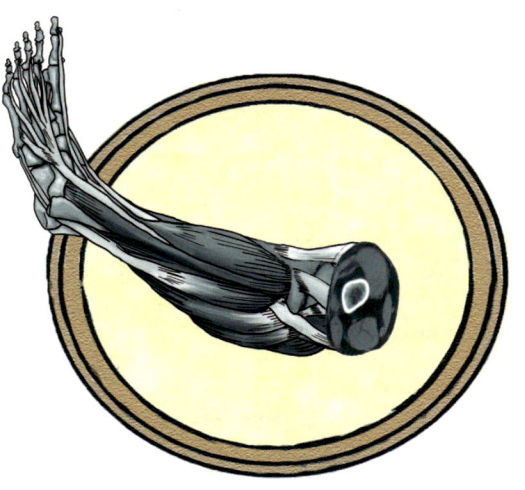

13. **Biceps femoris** (*M. biceps femoris*)

14. **Tendon of the short head of biceps femoris** (*Ten. biceps femoris, caput breve*)

15. **Iliotibial tract** (*Tractus iliotibialis*)

16. **Lateral head of the gastrocnemius** (*M.gastrocnemius caput laterale*)

1. **Patella** (*Patella*)

2. **Patellar tendon** (*Ten. patellae*)

3. **Pre-patellar bursa** (*Bursa subfascialis pre-patellaris*)

4. **Vastus medialis** (*M. vastus medialis*)

5. **Femur** (*Os femoris*)

6. **Popliteal vein** (*Vena poplitea*)

7. **Popliteal artery** (*Arteria poplitea*)

8. **Sartorius** (*M. sartorius*)

9. **Gracilis** (*M. gracilis*)

10. **Semimembranosus** (*M. semimembranosus*)

11. **Semitendinosus tendon** (*Ten. semitendinosus*)

12. **Tibial nerve** (*N. tibialis*)

V – Mid-Knee – Medial

In this section, the lower extremity has been sliced superior to the knee, and rotated to show the medial structures. The patellar ligament is at 12 o'clock, and below this, the femur is now a two-pronged lateral and medial condyle. In the space between these condyles the cruciate ligaments are seen crossing each other, the posterior ligament more medial, and heading for its distal attachment on the posterior aspect of the tibia. The medial collateral ligament and sartorius occupy the 2 and 3 o'clock positions. Just posterior to sartorius is the tendon of gracilis. The medial head of gastrocnemius is at 6 o'clock, and the tendon of semitendinosus occupies the postero-medial border of this muscle. A corresponding CT shows these structures radiographically.

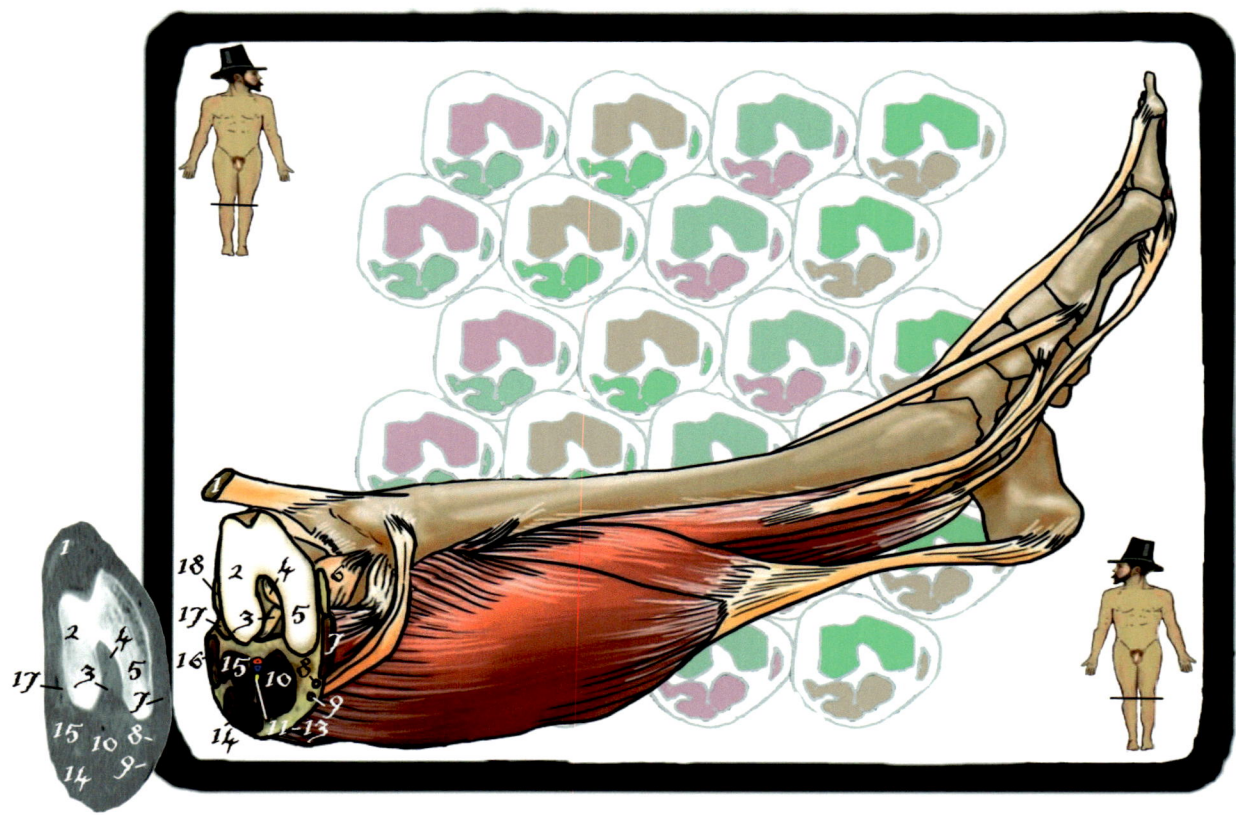

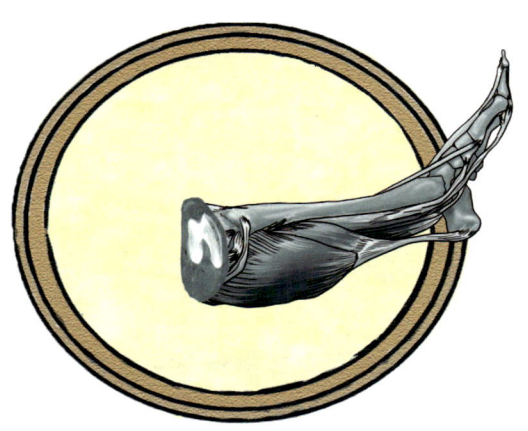

14. **Lateral head of the gastrocnemius** (*M. gastrocnemius, caput laterale*)

15. **Plantaris** (*M. plantaris*)

16. **Tendon of the short head of biceps femoris** (*Ten. biceps femoris, caput breve*)

17. **Lateral collateral ligament** (*Lig. collaterale laterale*)

18. **Iliotibial tract** (*Tractus iliotibialis*)

1. **Patellar tendon** (*Ten. patellae*)

2. **Lateral condyle of the femur** (*Condylus lateralis*)

3. **Anterior cruciate ligament** (*Lig. cruciatum anterius*) From crux, or cruciare, the Latin terms for a cross, or the verb to cross.

4. **Posterior cruciate ligament** (*Lig. cruciatum posterius*)

5. **Medial condyle of the femur** (*Condylus medialis*)

6. **Medial collateral ligament** (*Lig. collaterale mediale*) The term ligament is derived from the Latin liger, meaning to bind.

7. **Sartorius** (*M. sartorius*)

8. **Gracilis tendon** (*Ten. gracilis*)

9. **Semitendinosus tendon** (*Ten. semitendinosus*)

10. **Medial head of the gastrocnemius** (*M. gastrocnemius, caput mediale*) According to Skinner, the term is derived from γαστροκνήμια, a combination of the words calf and belly. The muscle was named by Hippocrates.

11. **Tibial nerve** (*N. tibialis*)

12. **Popliteal vein** (*Vena poplitea*)

13. **Popliteal artery** (*Arteria poplitea*)

VI – Mid-Knee – Lateral

Superior to the lateral condyle, the iliotibial tract is seen heading across the knee to the tibia. The cruciate ligaments may be seen, the anterior cruciate ligament sitting more medial than its posterior counterpart. Between 8 and 9 o'clock, the tendon of biceps femoris can be followed down to the lateral head of the fibula. Below the lateral condyle, plantaris sits above the lateral head of gastrocnemius. A corresponding CT shows these structures radiographically.

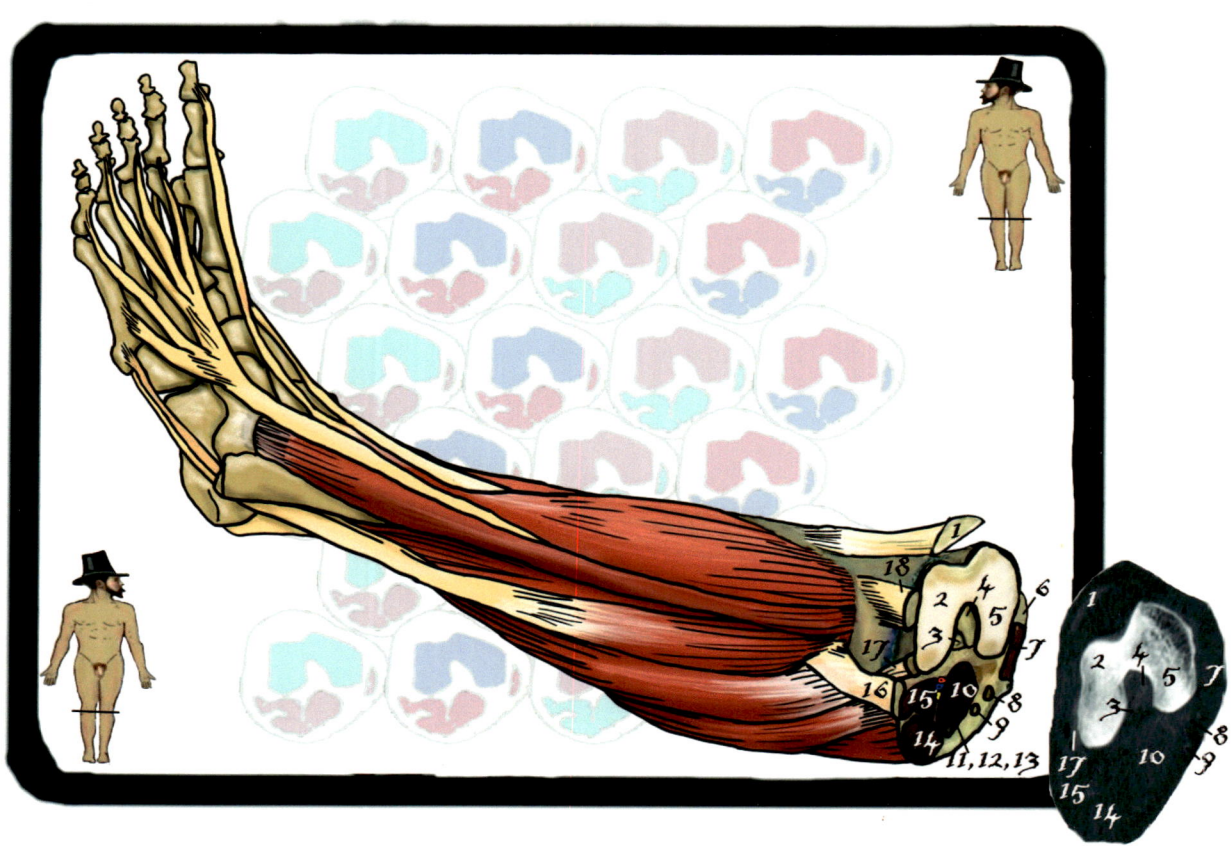

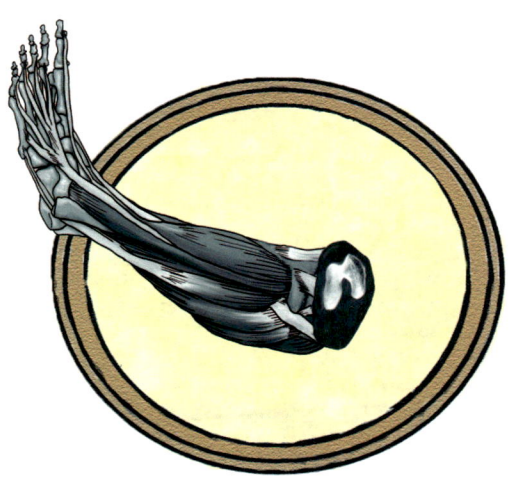

16. **Tendon of the short head of biceps femoris** (*Ten. biceps femoris, caput breve*)

17. **Lateral collateral ligament** (*Lig. collaterale laterale*)

19. **Iliotibial tract** (*Tractus iliotibialis*)

1. **Patellar tendon** (*Ten. patellae*)

2. **Lateral condyle of the femur** (*Condylus lateralis*)

3. **Anterior cruciate ligament** (*Lig. cruciatum anterius*)

4. **Posterior cruciate ligament** (*Lig. cruciatum posterius*)

5. **Medial condyle of the femur** (*Condylus medialis*)

6. **Medial collateral ligament** (*Lig. collaterale mediale*)

7. **Sartorius** (*M. sartorius*)

8. **Gracilis tendon** (*Ten. gracilis*)

9. **Semitendinosus tendon** (*Ten. semitendinosus*)

10. **Medial head of the gastrocnemius** (*M. gastrocnemius, caput mediale*)

11. **Tibial nerve** (*N. tibialis*)

12. **Popliteal vein** (*Vena poplitea*)

13. **Popliteal artery** (*Arteria poplitea*)

14. **Lateral head of the gastrocnemius** (*M. gastrocnemius, caput laterale*)

15. **Plantaris** (*M. plantaris*)

VII – Inferior Knee – Medial

In this section, the lower extremity has been sectioned through the inferior aspect of the knee, and rotated to show medial structures. The patella tendon is at 12 o'clock, and the distal ends of the femoral condyles are seen. The cruciate ligaments cross, with the posterior cruciate ligament more medial. Sartorius is at 3 o'clock, just below the medial collateral ligament. Beneath sartorius, the distal ends of gracilis and semitendinosus tendons are seen. At 6 o'clock sits the medial head of grastrocnemius. A corresponding CT shows these structures radiographically.

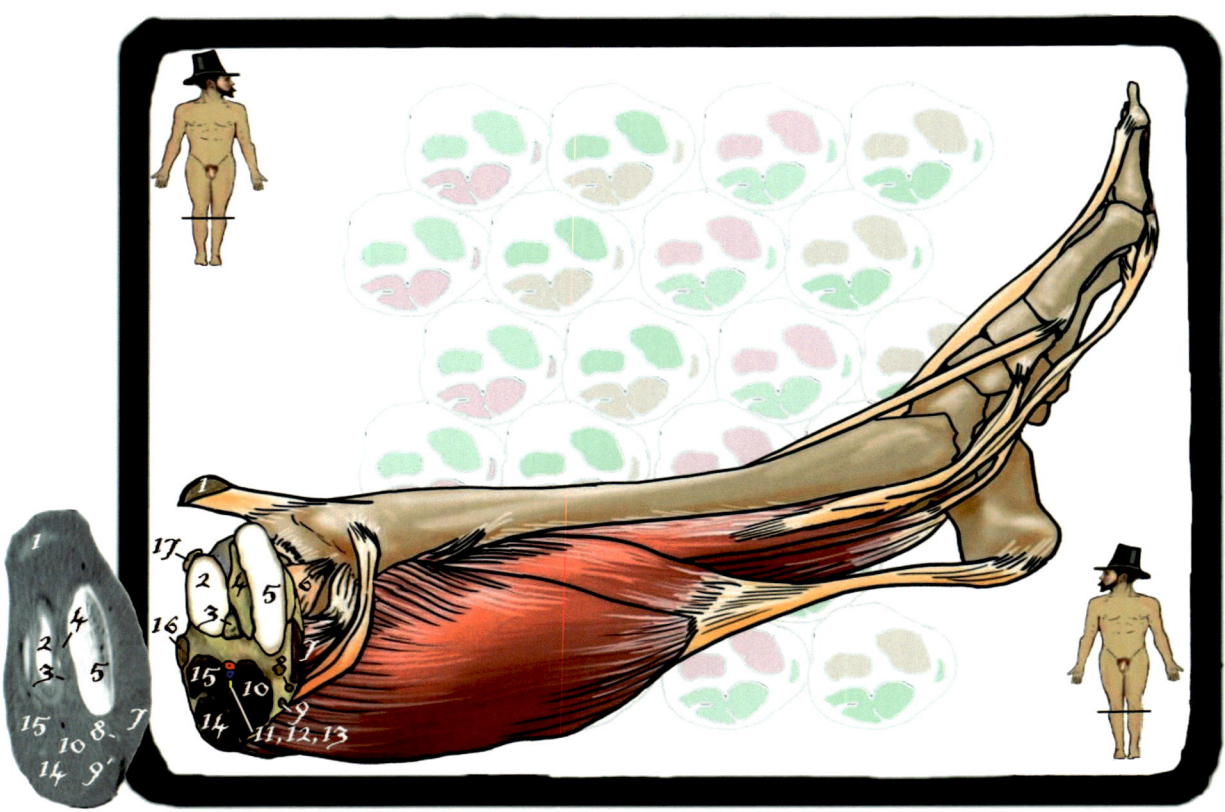

14. **Lateral head of the gastrocnemius** (*M. gastrocnemius, caput laterale*)

15. **Plantaris** (*M. plantaris*)

16. **Tendon of the short head of biceps femoris** (*Ten. biceps femoris, caput breve*)

17. **Iliotibial tract** (*Tractus iliotibialis*)

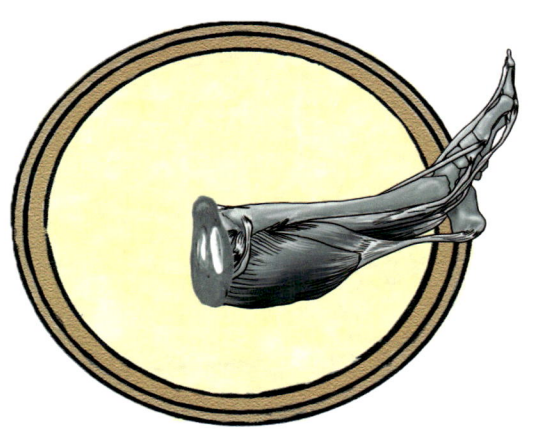

1. **Patellar tendon** (*Ten. patellae*)

2. **Lateral condyle of the femur** (*Condylus lateralis*)

3. **Anterior cruciate ligament** (*Lig. cruciatum anterius*)

4. **Posterior cruciate ligament** (*Lig. cruciatum posterius*)

5. **Medial condyle of the femur** (*Condylus medialis*)

6. **Medial collateral ligament** (*Lig. collaterale mediale*)

7. **Sartorius** (*M. sartorius*)

8. **Gracilis tendon** (*Ten. gracilis*)

9. **Semitendinosus tendon** (*Ten. semitendinosus*)

10. **Medial head of the gastrocnemius** (*M. gastrocnemius, caput mediale*)

11. **Tibial nerve** (*N. tibialis*)

12. **Popliteal vein** (*Vena poplitea*)

13. **Popliteal artery** (*Arteria poplitea*)

VIII – Inferior Knee – Lateral

In this section the lower extremity has been sectioned through the inferior aspect of the knee, and rotated to show lateral structures. Near the lateral condyle, the cruciate ligaments may be seen, the anterior ligament more lateral than the posterior ligament. Posterior to the lateral condyle is the belly of plantaris. Posterior to this muscle sits the lateral head of gastrocnemius. At 6 o'clock, between plantaris and the medial head of gastrocnemius, are the peroneal vessels and the tibial nerve. The biceps tendon can be followed from 9 o'clock to its attachment on the fibular head. A corresponding CT shows these structures radiographically.

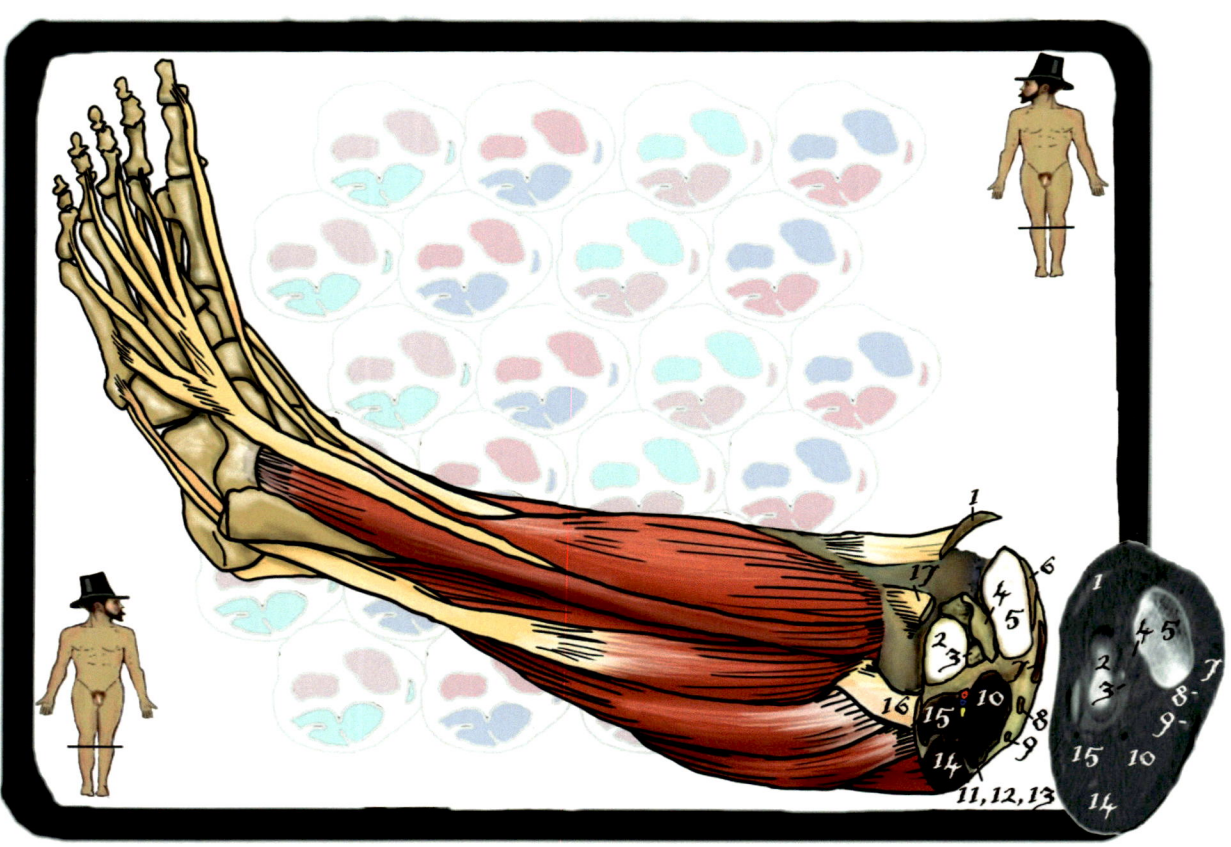

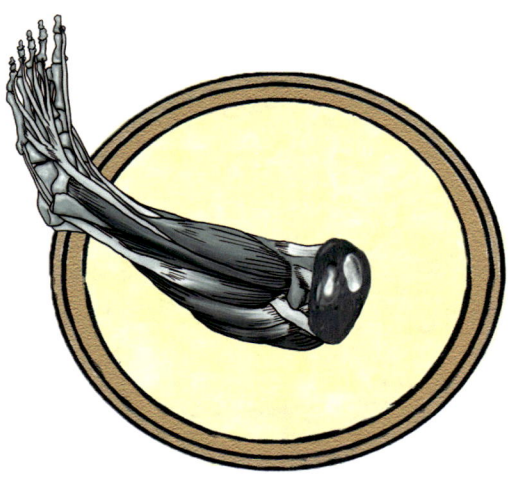

14. **Lateral head of the gastrocnemius** (*M. gastrocnemius, caput laterale*)

15. **Plantaris** (*M. plantaris*)

16. **Tendon of the short head of biceps femoris** (*Ten. biceps femoris, caput breve*)

17. **Iliotibial tract** (*Tractus iliotibialis*)

1. **Patellar tendon** (*Ten. patellae*)

2. **Lateral condyle of the femur** (*Condylus lateralis*)

3. **Anterior cruciate ligament** (*Lig. cruciatum anterius*)

4. **Posterior cruciate ligament** (*Lig. cruciatum posterius*)

5. **Medial condyle of the femur** (*Condylus medialis*)

6. **Medial collateral ligament** (*Lig. collaterale mediale*)

7. **Sartorius** (*M. sartorius*)

8. **Gracilis tendon** (*Ten. gracilis*)

9. **Semitendinosus tendon** (*Ten. semitendinosus*)

10. **Medial head of the gastrocnemius** (*M. gastrocnemius, caput mediale*)

11. **Tibial nerve** (*N. tibialis*)

12. **Popliteal vein** (*Vena poplitea*)

13. **Popliteal artery** (*Arteria poplitea*)

IX – Mid-Leg – Medial

The leg has been sliced through the mid-lower leg and rotated to show medial structures. At 12 o'clock is the tibia, medial to which sits flexor digitorum at 1 o'clock. The peroneal vessels and tibial nerve are seen between f. digitorum and tibialis posterior. The tendon of the latter muscle can be seen closer to the ankle joint. Next to f. digitorum is flexor hallucis longus. Soleus occupies a position from about 2 to 8 o'clock. The distal end of gastrocnemius is seen at 5 o'clock. A corresponding CT shows these structures radiographically.

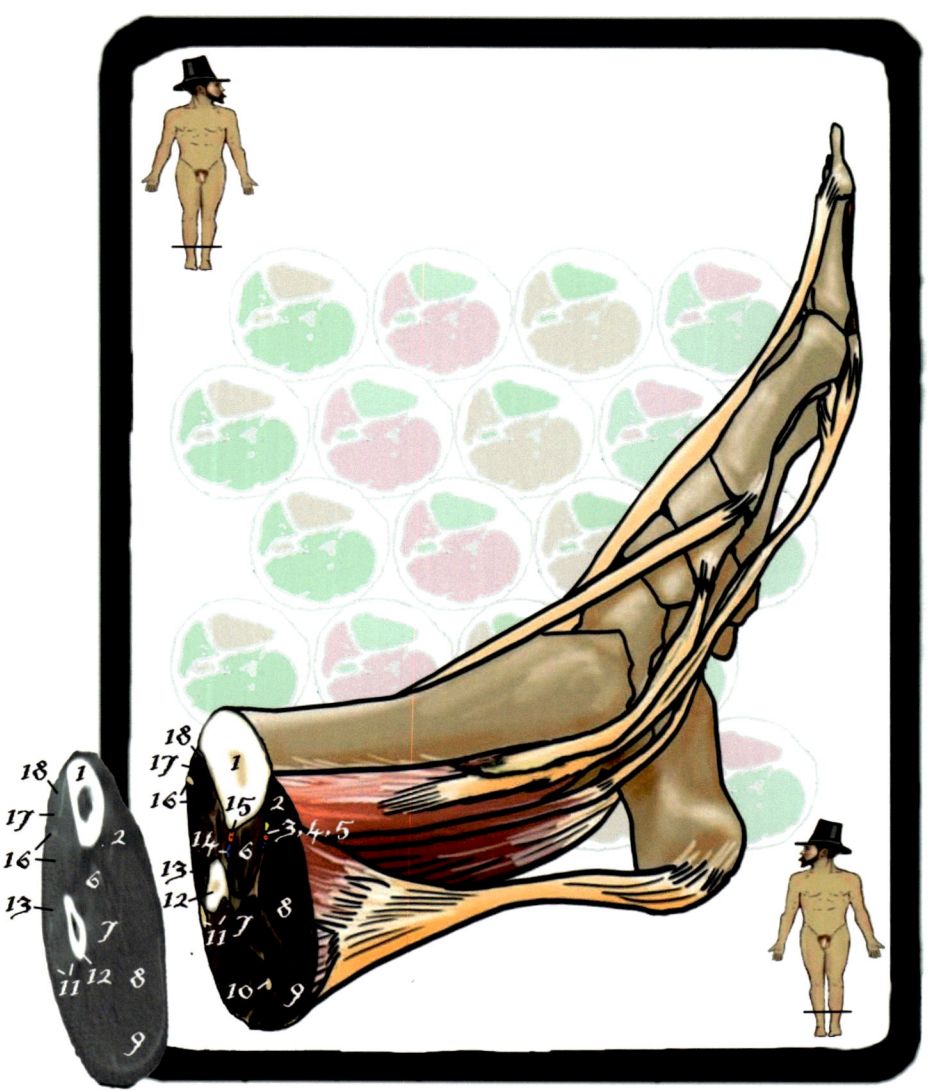

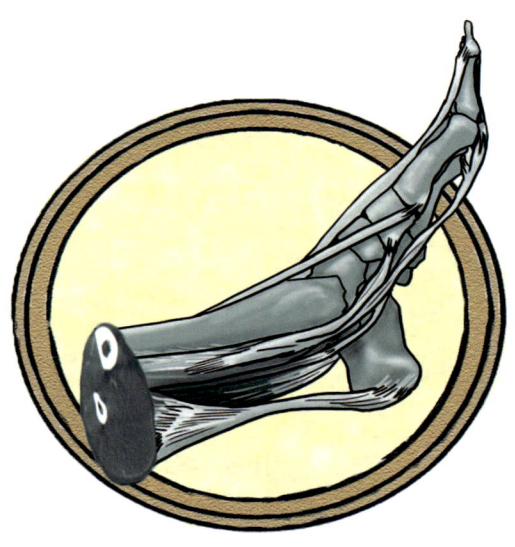

13. **Peroneus/fibularis brevis** (*M. peroneus/fibularis brevis*)

14. **Anterior tibial vein** (*Vena tibialis anterior*)

15. **Anterior tibial artery** (*Arteria tibialis anterior*)

16. **Extensor digitorum longus muscle and tendon** (*M. et ten. extensor digitorum longus*)

17. **Extensor hallucis longus** (*M. extensor hallucis longus*)

18. **Tibialis anterior** (*M. tibialis anterior*)

1. **Tibia** (*Tibia*) Derived from the Latin term for a flute, or tuba-like horn, the bone was named by Celsus in the 1st century.

2. **Flexor digitorum longus** (*M. flexor digitorum longus*)

3. **Tibial nerve** (*N. tibialis*)

4. **Peroneal vein** (*V. peroneale*)

5. **Peroneal artery** (*A. peroneale*)

6. **Tibialis posterior** (*M. tibialis posterior*)

7. **Flexor hallucis longus** (*M. flexor hallucis longus*)

8. **Soleus** (*M. soleus*) The name for this muscle, popularized by Riolan in the 17th century, refers to the sole, a fish whose shape the muscle was thought to resemble.

9. **Gastrocnemius** (*M. gastrocnemius*)

10. **Plantaris tendon** (*Ten. plantaris*)

11. **Peroneus/fibularis longus muscle and tendon** (*M. et ten. peroneus/fibularis longus*) Peroneus is an 18th century term derived from περον, meaning the pointed clasp of a buckle.

12. **Fibula** (*Fibula*) Named by Vesalius, the term is derived from the Latin term for a clasp, like those used to secure a toga.

X – Mid-Leg – Lateral

In this section, the lower extremity has been sectioned in the mid-part of the lower leg. At 12 o'clock is the tibia, lateral to which sits tibialis anterior. At 10 o'clock is extensor hallucis, and at 9 o'clock is extensor digitorum. The tendons of these muscles can be traced distally. Peroneus brevis and longus can also be seen at around 8 o'clock, and their tendons traced distally as well. A corresponding CT shows these structures radiographically.

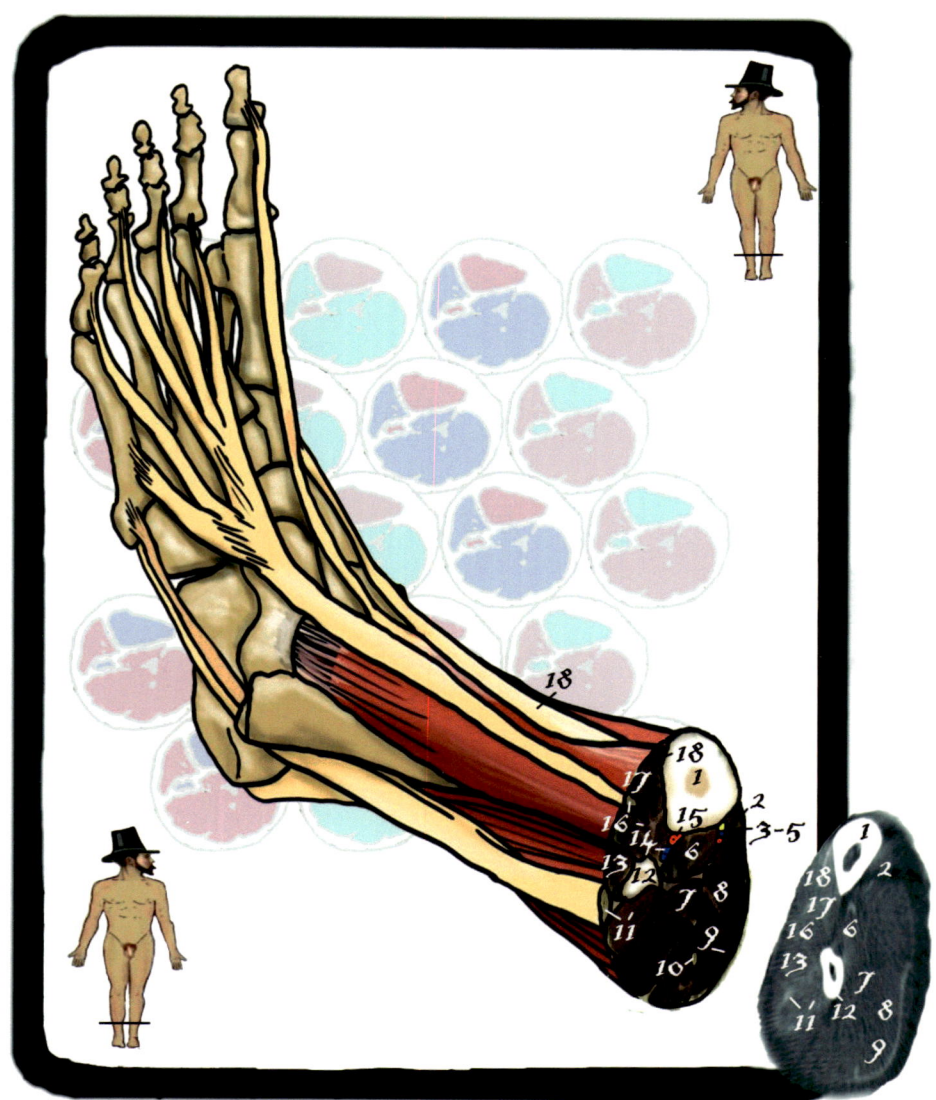

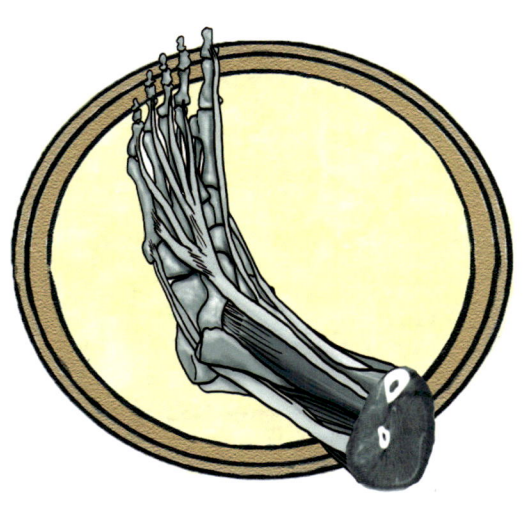

15. **Anterior tibial artery** (*Arteria tibialis anterior*)

16. **Extensor digitorum longus muscle and tendon** (*M. et ten. extensor digitorum longus*)

17. **Extensor hallucis longus** (*M. extensor hallucis longus*)

18. **Tibialis anterior** (*M. tibialis anterior*)

1. **Tibia** (*Tibia*)

2. **Flexor digitorum longus** (*M. flexor digitorum longus*)

3. **Tibial nerve** (*N. tibialis*)

4. **Peroneal vein** (*V. peroneale*)

5. **Peroneal artery** (*A. peroneale*)

6. **Tibialis posterior** (*M. tibialis posterior*)

7. **Flexor hallucis longus** (*M. flexor hallucis longus*)

8. **Soleus** (*M. soleus*)

9. **Gastrocnemius** (*M. gastrocnemius*)

10. **Plantaris tendon** (*Ten. plantaris*)

11. **Peroneus/fibularis longus muscle and tendon** (*M. et ten. peroneus/fibularis longus*)

12. **Fibula** (*Fibula*)

13. **Peroneus/fibularis brevis** (*M. peroneus/fibularis brevis*)

14. **Anterior tibial vein** (*Vena tibialis anterior*)

XI – Distal – Medial

In this section, the lower extremity has been sectioned at the tibiofibular joint, slightly superior to the ankle. Tibialis anterior tendon is seen at 12 o'clock. At 3 o'clock sits the tendon of tibialis posterior, while just below this at 4 o'clock is the tendon of flexor digitorum longus. At 5 o'clock is the remnant muscle belly and tendon of flexor hallucis longus. The tendons of fibularis longus and brevis are more lateral, and should not be associated with the belly of pollicis longus. The Achilles, or calcaneal, tendon is at 6 o'clock. A corresponding CT shows these structures radiographically.

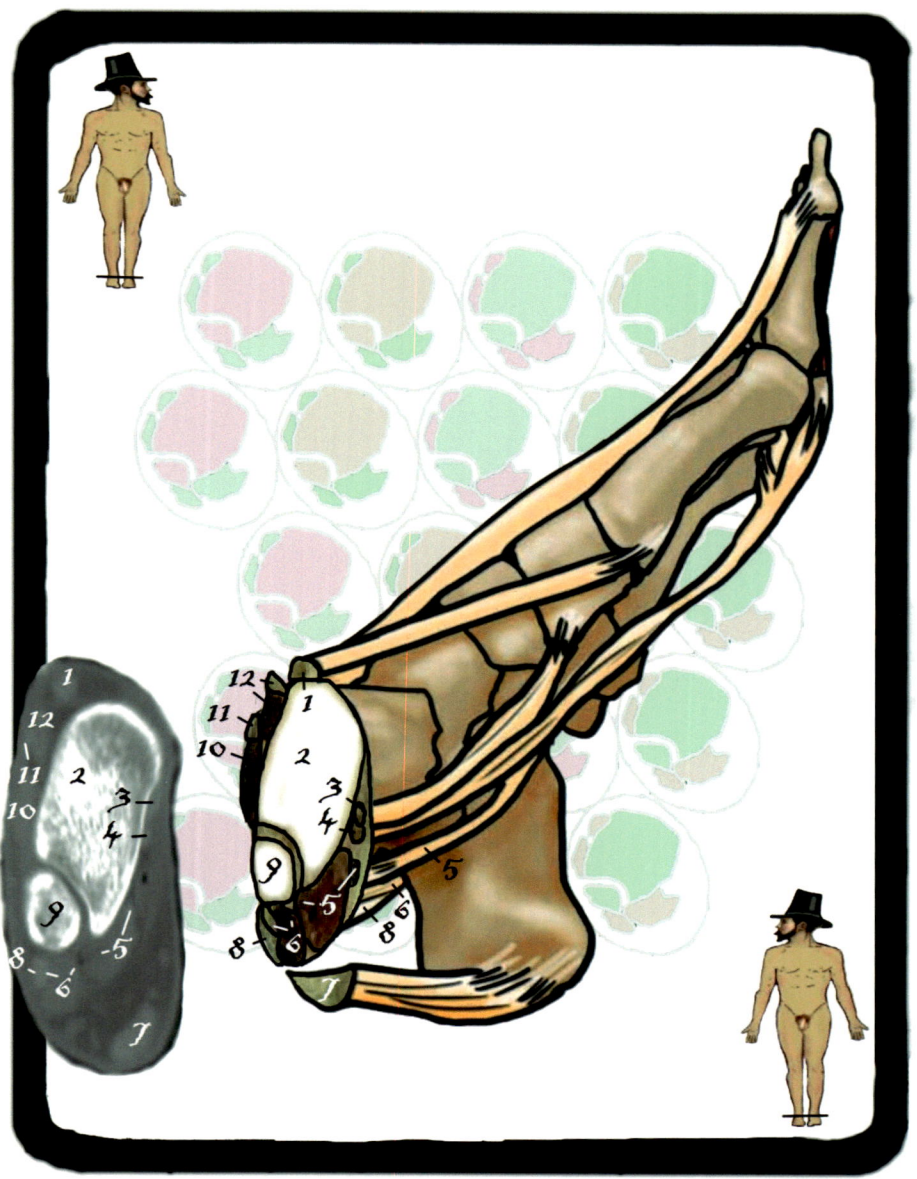

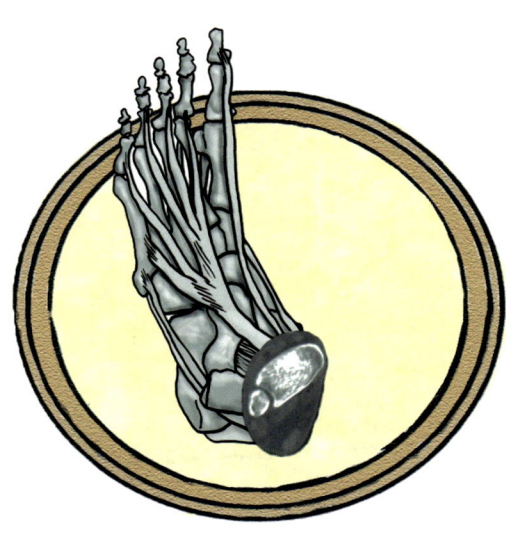

9. **Fibula** (*Fibula*)

10. **Extensor digitorum longus** (*M. extensor digitorum longus*)

11. **Extensor digitorum longus tendon** (*Ten. extensor digitorum longus*)

12. **Extensor hallucis longus** (*M. extensor hallucis longus*)

1. **Tibialis anterior tendon** (*Ten. tibialis anterior*)

2. **Tibia** (*Tibia*)

3. **Tibialis posterior tendon** (*Ten. tibialis posterior*)

4. **Flexor digitorum longus muscle and tendon** (*M. et ten. flexor digitorum longus*)

5. **Flexor hallucis longus muscle and tendon** (*M. ten. flexor hallucis longus*)

6. **Peroneus/fibularis longus brevis** (*M. peroneus/fibularis brevis*)

7. **Calcaneus/Achilles tendon** (*Tendo calcaneus*) The term tendon is derived from the Latin verb tendere, to stretch out, and was used by Homer. Although the Achilles Tendon—named for the mythological hero who, held by his heel, was dipped into the waters of the river Styx to make him invincible—was described by Hippocrates, the eponym was not used until the 17th century.

8. **Peroneus/fibularis longus tendon** (*Ten. peroneus/fibularis longus*)

XII – Distal Leg – Lateral

In this section, the lower extremity has been sectioned at the tibiofibular joint and rotated to show lateral structures. At 11 o'clock, the wispy ends of flexor hallucis longus can be seen converging into a tendon, and then traced out to its distal attachment on the great toe. At 9 and 10 o'clock, extensor digitorum longus can be seen, its muscle belly turning into tendons. At 7 o'clock, just posterior to the fibula, the tendons of fibularis longus and brevis are seen, and these may be followed inferiorly to the fifth metatarsal. A corresponding CT shows these structures radiographically.

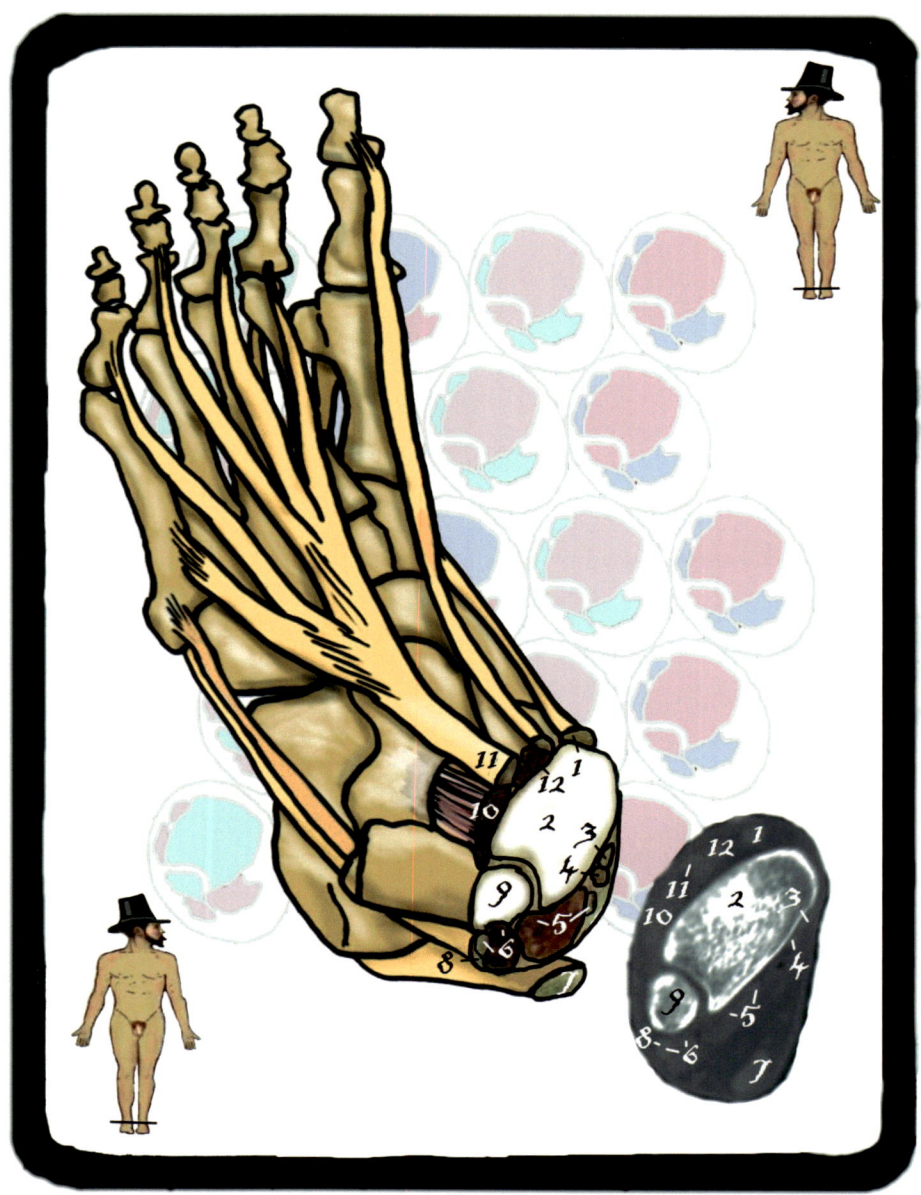

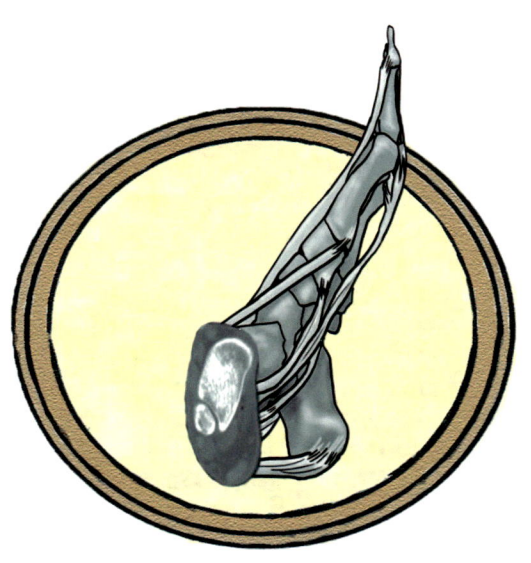

10. **Extensor digitorum longus** (*M. extensor digitorum longus*)

11. **Extensor digitorum longus tendon** (*Ten. extensor digitorum longus*)

12. **Extensor hallucis longus** (*M. extensor hallucis longus*)

1. **Tibialis anterior tendon** (*Ten. tibialis anterior*)

2. **Tibia** (*Tibia*)

3. **Tibialis posterior tendon** (*Ten. tibialis posterior*)

4. **Flexor digitorum longus tendon** (*Ten. flexor digitorum longus*)

5. **Flexor hallucis longus muscle and tendon** (*M. et ten. flexor hallucis longus*)

6. **Peroneus/fibularis longus brevis** (*M. peroneus/fibularis brevis*)

7. **Calcaneus/Achilles tendon** (*Tendo calcaneus*)

8. **Peroneus/fibularis longus tendon** (*Ten. peroneus/fibularis longus*)

9. **Fibula** (*Fibula*)